THE
PROBIOTICS
REVOLUTION

THE
PROBIOTICS
REVOLUTION

Dr Gary Huffnagle
with Sarah Wernick

Vermilion
LONDON

WORCESTERSHIRE COUNTY COUNCIL		
	647	
First publishe	Bertrams	02.10.07
Published in 20		
A	613.26	£12.99
Copyright		
Gary Huffnagle, PhD and S	WO	the

Gary Huffnagle, PhD and Sarah Wernick have asserted their right to be identified as the
authors of this Work in accordance with the Copyright, Design and Patents Act 1988

The Random House Group Limited Reg. No. 954009
Addresses for companies within the Random House Group can be found at
www.randomhouse.co.uk

A CIP catalogue record for this book is available from the British Library

The Random House Group Limited makes every effort to ensure that the papers used
in our books are made from trees that have been legally sourced from well-managed
and credibly certified forests. Our paper procurement policy can be found on

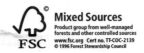

Mixed Sources
Product group from well-managed
forests and other controlled sources
www.fsc.org Cert no. TT-COC-2139
FSC © 1996 Forest Stewardship Council

Book design by Carol Malcolm Russo

Printed and bound in Great Britain by
Clays Ltd, St Ives Plc

ISBN 9780091922030

The Healing Foods Pyramid was created by Monica Myklebust, MD, and
Jenna Wunder, MPH, RD, at the University of Michigan Department of Family Medicine.
Excerpts are included in the book with the permission of copyright holders, the Regents of
the University of Michigan, Monica Myklebust, MD, and Jenna Wunder, MPH, RD.

Illustrations by Michigan Marketing and Design, University of Michigan. Quotation
from Alexander Fleming's Nobel Lecture copyright © 1945 by the Nobel Foundation,
reprinted with permission.

Copies are available at special rates for bulk orders.
Contact the sales development team on 020 7840 8487 for more information.

To buy books by your favourite authors and register for offers, visit
www.rbooks.co.uk

To Kathy, Erin and Ryan,
for all of their support and encouragement
throughout the intensive process
of turning my idea for a book into reality

ACKNOWLEDGEMENTS

This work is built on the shoulders of those who came before. It has been solidified by discussions and critiques with many colleagues in the medical sciences.

First of all, I want to acknowledge Mairi Noverr, PhD, for her extensive contributions to this project. First as a graduate student under my mentorship and then as a postdoctoral fellow, she has helped me explore the world of microbial interactions with their host. Our extensive conversations about probiotics and prebiotics have been invaluable for this book, which explains the positive role that our microflora plays in shaping our immune responses. I will always be indebted to her for her tireless efforts, dedication and enthusiasm in the laboratory, and will always cherish her belief and trust in me.

I would like to acknowledge all the members of my lab – current and past – for their dedication and enthusiasm. Their range of experience and expertise is wide – from freshman undergraduates through graduate students and postdoctoral fellows, and from research assistants to research associates to research faculty. But all have made invaluable contributions to our research. Their positive spirits have made the lab a dynamic, upbeat environment. This book is a testament to their accomplishments and I thank all of them from the bottom of my heart.

Many thanks as well to my mentors: Edwin Gaffney, PhD, Mary Lipscomb, MD, and Galen Toews, MD. When I was an undergraduate, Dr Gaffney and his lab provided me with my first research experience and fostered my interest in medical research. At a point when my interest might have waned, Dr Lipscomb and the members of her lab reignited my excitement. She also gave me tremendous encouragement and advice for which I will be forever grateful. Dr Toews has been not only my Division Chief in Pulmonary Medicine for the past fourteen years, but has also been my mentor, research partner and friend during my career at the University of Michigan. I'm especially indebted to him for his support when I decided to test the off-the-wall idea that the microbiology of the gut might provide new insights into diseases of the lungs.

My appreciation to my fellow faculty members in the Pulmonary Division at the University of Michigan Medical School. Their collegiality, advice and support have made my tenure in the division both enjoyable and productive. I also want to thank all the other members of the division staff, with a special thank you to Cat Meyer, who has been there since the beginning. Together, they have made it feel like home for the past fourteen years. My appreciation as well to my other colleagues in the Department of Internal Medicine, especially my Department Chair, Dr Marc Lippman, for his strong support of my research and educational endeavours.

I feel fortunate to have two departmental 'homes' at the University of Michigan. I'm grateful to my great colleagues in the Department of Microbiology and Immunology for their support and advice through the years. I also want to thank the department administrative staff for their warmth and their assistance.

I am indebted to Dr Juneann Murphy and Dr Thomas Kozel for their counselling and mentorship throughout these many years. Their scientific and career advice has been invaluable and I appreciate it. I also want to thank, in aggregate, my other colleagues in the field of medical mycology. They are a truly supportive group. In addition, I want to acknowledge the Immunology Graduate Program at the University of Texas Southwestern Medical School – an incredible programme with a dedicated faculty and great friends who have gone on to become great colleagues.

The National Institute of Allergy and Infectious Diseases; the National Heart, Lung, and Blood Institute; the Parker B. Francis Fellowship Program and the Burroughs-Wellcome Fund have provided generous support of the research in my laboratory over the years, for which I am most grateful. Through this work, some of which is described in the book, my colleagues and I have examined the role of our microflora in health and disease.

This book is a joint effort with freelance writer Sarah Wernick. Both of us would like to express our gratitude to the people who have helped us. Many thanks to our wonderful agent, Ted Weinstein, for his dedication in bringing this project to fruition. His energy and attention to detail have helped us from start to finish. Working with Toni Burbank, editor extraordinaire at Bantam Dell, has been a joy. We appreciate her guidance, her enthusiastic support – and most of all, her extensive and marvellously helpful comments on the manuscript. Our thanks to associate editor Julie Will for her valuable assistance and unfailing good cheer.

Our appreciation to the talented writers who provided valuable comments on the book proposal and individual chapters: Anita

Bartholomew, Pat McNees, Sally Wendkos Olds and Barbara Sofer. We're particularly grateful to William Lockeretz, PhD, who painstakingly reviewed the entire manuscript for clarity as well as for technical and grammatical accuracy.

We would also like to thank the individuals who provided material for this book. The following people agreed to speak with us about their experiences with probiotics: Michael Cabana, MD, of the University of California, San Francisco; John Kao, MD, of the University of Michigan; Marcelle Pick, RNC, OB/GYN NP, of Women to Women in Yarmouth, Maine; Dana Reed, MS, CNS, CDN, of ReedNutrition.com; David Rubin, MD, of the University of Chicago and his patient, Mordechai Eliezer Smith; Jay Sandweiss, DO, of Ann Arbor, Michigan; Jeff Terrell, MD, of the University of Michigan and Vince Young, MD, PhD, of Michigan State University.

Special appreciation to Monica Myklebust, MD, and Jenna Wunder, MPH, RD, of the University of Michigan, creators of the Healing Foods Pyramid, who have kindly allowed us to quote their work extensively.

Our warm thanks to Mary Ellen Sanders, executive director of the International Scientific Association for Probiotics and Prebiotics, who generously offered detailed critical comments on the manuscript. We're also grateful to Michael T Murray, ND, for his very helpful suggestions. However, I want to emphasise that the views expressed in this book are my own, and may not agree with theirs in all respects.

I also want to acknowledge the ever-cheerful staff at Angelo's – my favourite place to enjoy a hot cup of dietary phenol-loaded beverage and contemplate our explorations into the unseen world of the microflora.

Finally, my personal thanks to my family: to my mom and dad for their support of their perpetual-student son and for that birthday present – many, many years ago – of my first microscope, and to my brothers, sisters-in-law, brother-in-law, father-in-law, nephews and niece for all their encouragement over the years.

Thank you all for your enthusiasm about my book. Most of all, a heartfelt thank you to my wife, Kathy, and to my children, Erin and Ryan. I appreciate their patience while I worked long hours on this project. I also want to thank them for all their help in reading and listening to this book as it was being written – and especially for their never-ending excitement about it. Particular thanks to my children for being willing 'test subjects' as we tried out the recipes and eating plans that are now in this book, including a few recipes that didn't make it!

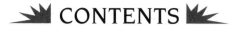

CONTENTS

PART THREE
Promoting Microbial Balance: What You Can Do

THE
PROBIOTICS
REVOLUTION

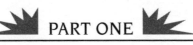

PART ONE

The Promise of Probiotics

*Natural forces within us are the
true healers of disease.*

— HIPPOCRATES

CHAPTER ONE

Our Silent Partners
for Good Health

When I was five years old, I received my first lesson in microbiology from a paper cup advert on TV. It showed magnified images of bug-like microbes, followed by a horrifying picture of a family's shared, bacteria-laden drinking glass in the bathroom. My health-conscious mother subsequently banished shared glasses and installed paper cup dispensers. Thus I learnt that all bacteria are bad and that we must avoid them to stay healthy.

Now that I spend my days (and many nights) tracking down the secrets of microbes, I know that none of that is true. In fact, some bacteria – called probiotics – are not only beneficial to our health, but actually essential. The term 'probiotics' comes from the Greek: *pro*, meaning 'promoting' and *biotic*, meaning 'life'. The word is sometimes used in a limited way, referring only to a few specific types of beneficial microbes contained in probiotic supplements or added to food. (See Notes at the end of the book.) But I prefer a broader definition – one that also includes the friendly microbes that normally live in our digestive tracts and that are naturally found in fermented foods, such as yoghurt, aged cheese and certain pickles.

The probiotic population in our digestive tract includes permanent residents, as well as tourists arriving via capsules or food. New research is revealing that that population often isn't large enough for optimal health. As a result, other bacteria can proliferate, creating an imbalance. Obviously, this affects how well our digestive system functions. But we're learning that the impact goes far beyond that. Probiotics are vital for our immune system, too. They actually send signals to the immune system that reduce destructive overreactions, including inflammation. This means that insufficiencies affect immune responses – and therefore every aspect of our health.

Though our bodies don't always contain enough probiotics, we can easily solve that problem. All it takes is increasing our consumption of certain healthy foods (many are probably in your diet already) and perhaps taking some readily available nutritional supplements, which need to be carefully selected. Best of all, these measures aren't risky. The effective foods taste good – and you'll begin to see benefits within weeks. If your diet is already healthy, you've made an excellent start. However, as this book will explain, there is much more you can do. And it doesn't have to happen all at once, because every little bit helps.

A NEW ESSENTIAL FOOD GROUP

Probiotics protect us in two ways. One is to compete successfully with potentially harmful microbes in our digestive tract, also known as the gut. That doesn't mean killing all of them. Rather, probiotics lower their population enough so that we're much less vulnerable to intestinal disorders and disease. Anyone who suffers chronic digestive problems knows that a healthy gut is essential to well-being – and sometimes maddeningly elusive.

Perhaps even more important, probiotics help the immune system to function properly. Our immune system acts like a police force, protecting us from germs. But if it overreacts, it can be the cause of disease rather than the cure. A trigger-happy immune system may discharge its potent weapons against harmless substances – dust, cat dander, eggs, peanuts – thereby producing allergic responses. These reactions are always uncomfortable and sometimes are severe enough to be life-threatening. An unrestrained immune system can even turn against our own cells, causing autoimmune disorders, such as ulcerative colitis, Crohn's disease and rheumatoid arthritis.

We can increase the probiotic population of our intestinal tract by consuming foods and supplements that contain these beneficial microbes. But we also must provide them with a hospitable place to live. Not surprisingly, our intestinal environment is shaped by what we eat. Certain foods, including products high in refined sugar, encourage the growth of harmful microbes. But other food components – called 'prebiotics' – strengthen probiotics. The first prebiotic to be discovered was a special type of fibre. Indeed, the usual use of the term focuses on this type of fibre exclusively. (See Notes.) But we're beginning to learn that other nutrients promote probiotics, too. In this book, I define prebiotics more broadly, including not only additional types of fibre, but also antioxidants, as well as certain proteins and fats, that help friendly microbes to thrive in our body.

It's not a coincidence that the list of prebiotics features items we already know are good for us. Most people know that foods rich in fibre and antioxidants – such as fruit, vegetables and whole grains – have a wide range of beneficial health benefits. I'm convinced that their underappreciated role as prebiotics helps explain why.

To me, probiotics and prebiotics aren't optional additions to our diet. They're an essential food group, one that provides nutrients just as important to our health as vitamins and minerals. This vital food group is missing from current nutrition recommendations. But I expect that omission to be corrected in the near future.

EXTRAORDINARY BENEFITS FROM ORDINARY FOODS

Medical scientists searching for new ways to optimise immune responses have found an effective solution in the supermarket. New evidence shows that probiotics can prevent and treat serious chronic illnesses. Below, I'll give you a preview. But we're also learning that probiotics ward off many minor problems that occasionally strike all of us, even if we're in apparently excellent health.

A fascinating Swedish study, published in *Environmental Health* in 2005, focused on 181 healthy men and women aged 18 to 65, all of them employed by the same company. Half were chosen at random to receive special straws that delivered a daily dose of probiotics as they sipped a beverage of their choice. The others were given look-alike straws containing no probiotics. For eighty days, participants used the straws and kept health diaries, recording any respiratory or gastrointestinal symptoms that caused them to call in ill.

During the study period, 26 per cent of those with the ordinary straws took time off from work because of gastrointestinal or respiratory illness. In contrast, only 16 per cent of the workers who received the probiotic required sick leave, a reduction of more than one-third. Other recent findings confirm that probiotics can prevent infectious disease (or at least speed up recovery). What's more, these striking benefits come without any adverse side effects.

The potential benefits of probiotics for those who suffer from chronic diseases are so extraordinary that they can sound like the claims that snake oil salesmen used to make at carnivals. But here at the University of Michigan Medical Center, as well as at other leading medical schools in the United States and abroad, research breakthroughs are bringing together the fields of microbiology, immunology, nutrition and physiology as never before. This collaboration has produced findings – some just emerging from the laboratory and not yet published – that are difficult to believe at first. In Part 2 of the book, I'll describe this work in more detail. Here's a sample:

Digestive Disorders: Diarrhoea, Inflammatory Bowel Disease, Irritable Bowel Syndrome and More

Digestive problems are a chronic private agony for millions and millions of people – and nearly all of us experience occasional unpleasant episodes. Difficulties can occur when the probiotic bacteria in our intestines are unable to compete with an onslaught of harmful bacteria.

Probiotics are now used to prevent or treat diarrhoea due to antibiotic treatment, infections, chemotherapy, radiation therapy or the unfamiliar microbes encountered in foreign travel. Many gastrointestinal specialists prescribe probiotic therapy for irritable bowel syndrome. Other common digestive problems that don't involve the immune system may respond to probiotics, too; one example is lactose intolerance.

Immune system malfunctions are responsible for chronic digestive problems that involve inflammation. One example is inflammatory bowel disease (IBD), a group of closely related diseases – including ulcerative colitis and Crohn's disease – in which the immune system overreacts to normal intestinal microbes, causing inflammation and ulcers (open sores). Several clinical trials – carefully controlled medical studies involving hundreds of patients – have found that probiotics show great promise for the treatment of IBD.

Allergies, Eczema, Asthma and Related Conditions

Allergic reactions, we now know, are caused when the immune system overreacts to harmless substances. Just within the past few years, we've discovered that probiotic bacteria can control these over-reactions. Exciting studies from Finland have found that when pregnant or breastfeeding women take probiotics, their babies are significantly less likely to suffer from eczema. This inflammatory skin reaction affects five million people in Britain, causing severe itching.

Now probiotics are under intense investigation as an allergy treatment. Currently, millions of allergy sufferers must choose between uncomfortable symptoms and significant side effects from medication. I'm confident that probiotic therapies, which rarely involve such problems, will resolve that dilemma.

Still another promising line of research involves asthma, a chronic condition in which the airways are inflamed and narrowed. People who suffer from asthma face terrifying attacks that can be triggered by allergies, exercise or adverse weather conditions. During an asthma attack, the airways narrow to the point where a person has difficulty breathing and could even die. Since asthma involves an inappropriate immune response, including inflammation, there's excellent reason to hope that probiotics could help.

Yeast Infections

Most yeast infections are caused by *Candida albicans,* a yeast that's normally kept in check by the probiotic *Lactobacillus* and other microbes that live in our intestines. But this natural defence may not always work. For example, hormonal changes, stress and a poor diet can predispose a woman to vaginal yeast infections. Or the problem may be antibiotic treatment, which doesn't harm yeasts but does kill their microbial competitors, allowing yeasts to proliferate.

Alternative medicine has long treated yeast infections by adding yoghurt or probiotic supplements to the diet; yoghurt is also a common folk remedy. Preliminary research suggests that certain probiotics are indeed effective.

Autoimmune Diseases

Autoimmune diseases are among the most baffling and disabling of conditions. We've identified more than eighty such diseases, including rheumatoid arthritis, type 1 diabetes, lupus and psoriasis. These conditions are not caused by some external enemy, but by our own immune system. Instead of protecting us, an overreactive immune system mistakes our own cells for harmful microbes and attacks them. For example, in rheumatoid arthritis, the erroneous target is the cells that make up our joints; in type 1 diabetes, it's the insulin-producing cells of the pancreas.

Probiotic bacteria have enormous potential to help, because they signal the immune system to show restraint. Scientists are just beginning to investigate how they might prevent or treat autoimmune diseases. One example: recent studies in laboratory animals highly susceptible to type 1 diabetes suggest that probiotics can actually prevent the condition.

Cardiovascular Disease, Obesity, Cancer and More

As our understanding of inflammation and the immune system expands, new possibilities emerge for probiotics. Because scientific attention to probiotics has just begun, many pieces of the puzzle are still missing. Nevertheless, a picture is developing as evidence accumulates. And support for this research is expanding rapidly. The National Institutes of Health has begun to fund research on probiotics, investigating their value in preventing or treating allergies, asthma, inflammatory bowel disease and other conditions.

Keep your eyes open! I expect you'll see many news stories about probiotics as we learn more about the health benefits of these remarkable bacteria. Meanwhile, here are a few intriguing examples of what's on the horizon:

Cardiovascular Disease

In the past decade, our whole approach to cardiovascular disease has changed drastically. The focus has moved from cholesterol to inflammation, which – we now realise – plays a major role in the arterial narrowing that leads to heart attacks and strokes.

Obesity

Could probiotics possibly combat obesity? We already know from the livestock industry that animals gain weight faster when their feed contains antibiotics, drugs that destroy probiotics. Very recent preliminary research suggests that changing the bacterial populations in the human gut could have the same effect, thereby contributing to obesity.

Colorectal Cancer

All of us are exposed to carcinogens (cancer-causing substances); our body may develop abnormal cells as a result. But we have defences to protect ourselves. For example, microbes in the intestines help ward off colorectal cancer by breaking down carcinogens in food to make them harmless. Also, the immune system – if it's functioning properly – recognises abnormal cells and destroys them. Scientists now speculate that boosting probiotic bacteria could help the body ward off colorectal cancer naturally, and perhaps prevent other cancers, too.

Tooth Decay and Gum Disease

Harmful bacteria can grow in the mouth, producing tooth decay and gum disease. A preliminary study from Japan has already found that people who eat plain yoghurt have lower rates of tooth decay than those who don't. And clinical trials are under way to see if probiotics can help prevent gum disease.

Fibromyalgia and Chronic Fatigue Syndrome

Medical researchers don't agree on the cause of these disabling diseases, whose symptoms can be described as a chronic flu. An emerging theory is that they are linked to the immune system and changes in the gut's bacterial population. Though we're a long way from having research findings to confirm this, some people report that their symptoms have been relieved by probiotics.

Autism

Autism, a condition involving unsociable and other abnormal behaviour, is on the rise. Among the many possible reasons, some experts believe, is the widespread use of antibiotics and the resulting changes in intestinal microbes. Clinical trials in England have suggested that probiotic supplements can help those autistic children whose symptoms developed after taking antibiotics and experiencing persistent diarrhoea.

WHY IS THIS A REVOLUTION?

Since the earliest microscopes were developed, in the late 1600s and early 1700s, we've known that microbes inhabit our body. But for three centuries their role in disease was not fully appreciated. In the late 1800s, Louis Pasteur and other scientists developed the germ theory, the then-revolutionary idea that disease is caused by microbes. Thanks to the germ theory, medical researchers began to identify the microbes that caused such killer diseases as bacterial pneumonia and tuberculosis, and they developed medications that destroyed them. Antibiotics were so extraordinarily successful in fighting diseases caused by germs that their widespread use, starting at the end of the Second World War, qualifies as another medical revolution.

However, from the 1960s onwards, there's been a dramatic rise in diseases and chronic conditions for which there is no obvious germ-based cause. Asthma is just one example: it's not identified with any germ, it's not infectious and its incidence has soared in the past four decades.

Scientists began to notice these puzzling changes in the late 1980s, as scattered reports pointed to increases in asthma and allergies. But more recently, new knowledge has revolutionised how we think about the microbes within us. We've discovered that they can improve immune system functioning, preventing or controlling chronic conditions and diseases that the germ theory doesn't satisfactorily explain.

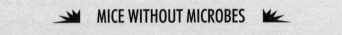

MICE WITHOUT MICROBES

What would life be like without the community of microbes that live in our gut? We can make educated guesses by looking at mice and other laboratory animals that are raised to be microbe-free. Only a few labs in the country, including those at the University of Michigan, can create and maintain these remarkable creatures. They have taught us much about the role of the digestive tract microbes in health and disease.

We begin by treating normal pregnant mice with antibiotics. The pups are delivered via Caesarean to avoid contamination in the birth canal. They're raised in sterile housing and fed sterile food and water; the air they breathe is sterilised, too. As a result, they have none of the digestive tract microbes normally found in mice. Future generations of these mice are born into this microbe-free world.

You might guess that microbe-free mice would be unusually healthy. But that's not true. Their immune system doesn't function properly. Consequently, if these mice are exposed to germs, they're abnormally susceptible to illness.

This role is so fundamental to our health that I now think of the microbes in our intestines as an organ, comparable in its effects and importance to other major organs such as the heart, lungs and kidneys. The key role of this 'organ' is to enable us to coexist with all the potentially harmful microbes we encounter in everyday life. If it can't perform properly, we lose the ability to remain healthy – and sometimes even to survive – in the normal world around us.

I'm so excited about the potential of probiotics that I talk about them to anyone who will listen. When I speak with a friend or colleague who's familiar with complementary or integrative medicine – or with someone from Europe, where probiotics are much better known and more widely used than they are in the United States – they often laugh and say, 'I know that' or 'My GP routinely recommends probiotics.' Sometimes they're puzzled that I'm describing this as a 'revolution'.

Complementary and integrative medicine has always empha-sised balance and the importance of looking at the whole body, not just the part with a troubling symptom. Healthcare specialists recognise that small differences in this balance can produce systemic effects. As a result, they often focus on wellness – building good health over time in a natural way, rather than rushing in with medical big guns only after we become ill. When I read the latest studies about probiotics in prestigious medical journals, I often marvel at the wisdom of Chinese doctors from centuries ago, who somehow knew that the intestines were not merely a digestive organ, but the centre of health and well-being.

What's new now is the contribution offered by controlled laboratory and clinical research. We're not only confirming that probiotics promote good health; we're also discovering which bacterial strains are most effective for particular problems. And as we begin to understand why they work, we're coming up with an even wider range of possible applications. What's truly revolutionary is that such safe, natural substances may be able to address some of our most prevalent, baffling and debilitating conditions.

Our knowledge is expanding rapidly as probiotics become the target of intense medical research. For years there had been a trickle of scientific articles on the subject, maybe half a dozen to a dozen annually. But the trickle became a flood. The number soared from 14 in 1995 to approximately 700 in 2005 – a 50-fold increase in just a decade! Scientific interest was stronger in Europe at first; many of the studies described in the book originated in other countries. But American researchers are becoming active in this area, and awareness is spreading to healthcare providers as well as to the public. They are beginning to realise that microbes in our digestive tract have profound effects on our health. The probiotics revolution has begun.

MY JOURNEY TO PROBIOTICS

By the 1960s, when I was a kid, America had already conquered many public health problems of the past. Behind this victory was an understanding of germs and nearly a century of advances in medical microbiology. Public hygiene had improved with better sewage disposal, water treatment and infection-control measures, such as quarantining highly infectious patients. Indoor plumbing gradually replaced the outhouse and the chamber pot. Thanks to all these changes, cholera and typhoid became rare.

Polio had been the scourge of my parents' childhoods. During summer – polio season – they had been forbidden to swim in streams, ponds or pools for fear of infection. My father's cousin Rex had been stricken as a child. Though he survived, his leg atrophied, requiring him to wear a brace and special shoes with extra-thick soles. But now vaccines protected my brothers and me from polio, as well as from smallpox, measles and mumps.

The war against infectious disease had recently acquired another powerful weapon: the miracle drugs called antibiotics.

The first, penicillin, became widely available after the Second World War, and many others soon joined it. During my childhood, doctors commonly prescribed antibiotics for colds, sore throats and earaches. I swallowed numerous antibiotic tablets to treat strep throat and bronchitis. My father's stepbrother, Jimmy, had died in 1942 at the age of 12 from an infection caused by a ruptured appendix. Every time my brothers and I heard the story about Uncle Jimmy and his tragic death, my parents would add the footnote: 'Jimmy wouldn't have died if he had been treated with antibiotics.'

No one realised that as we were winning the battle against infectious diseases, other enemies were gathering strength. The first to be noticed – because they affected children – were allergies and asthma. I was an early victim of both emerging epidemics.

Asthma attacks came without warning, often in the middle of the night. I'd wake up suddenly, gasping for breath. It felt as though I was trying to breathe through a narrow straw. No matter how hard I tried, I couldn't get enough air. Panicked, I'd run to wake my mother. 'Mum! I can't breathe!' She'd jump out of bed and race to the bathroom for my theophylline tablets and a glass of water. I'd gulp down the pills. Then we'd sit and wait for them to take effect. These episodes terrified my parents and me. Although I got extra attention, not to mention the privilege of sleeping in the one air-conditioned room in the house, I hated being the only kid I knew who had asthma.

My respiratory allergies – caused by mould spores, dust and many other common substances – were even worse, because they constantly interfered with my life. After school, instead of joining my friends to play every day, I went to the doctor's surgery two or three times a week for allergy injections. I spent most of July and August in the air-conditioned room, away from the high pollen content of a summer day in central Pennsylvania. In the 1970s, we didn't have computers, video games, VCRs or instant messaging. Being banished from the outdoors seemed terrible. In the winter, real Christmas trees were banned from the house after we learnt that my annual extremely severe holiday 'cold' was actually an allergic response to the fragrant evergreens that had once adorned our family room.

Allergies and asthma put an end to my childhood dream of being a baseball star (or maybe it was my inability to hit a curveball). But they undoubtedly inspired my interest in medical research. The world of the unseen fascinated me. Astronauts had just begun to explore outer space. In my eyes, microbiology was – and remains – an equally exciting exploration of an uncharted living world, an 'inner space'.

In college, at Penn State University in Pennsylvania, I studied microbiology. After college, I headed down to Southwestern Medical School in Texas to study immunology, which focuses on the body's immune system. Our professors taught us that the number one job of the immune system was to kill germs.

No one in school talked about probiotics. But I had read about these helpful microbes in a biography of the Nobel Prize-winning immunologist Ilya Mechnikov. In the early 1900s, Mechnikov turned his interests to health and longevity studies. He became intrigued by the long life spans of Bulgarian peasants. Despite their poverty and rural isolation, they lived longer than any other group in Europe, even the most privileged.

Mechnikov discovered that their diet was unusually rich in fermented foods, including yoghurt. He identified the bacterium used to ferment these foods and named it *Lactobacillus bulgaricus*. These microbes, he speculated, were responsible for the remarkably long lives of the Bulgarians. Based on his research, Mechnikov predicted that beneficial bacteria could be far more important to human health than disease-causing bacteria.

Eight decades later, around the time I entered graduate school, the National Institutes of Health was not funding projects that explored Mechnikov's hypothesis. However, a new understanding of our immune system was taking hold among immunologists.

Apparently, the immune system not only *protected against* disease; it could also *cause* disease.

Researchers had just demonstrated that respiratory allergy symptoms were not caused by the allergen. Rather, the immune system itself was the culprit. Instead of recognising substances like pollen or mould as harmless, the immune system of an allergic individual reacted as if they were dangerous germs. The sinuses and airways became inflamed, bringing in white blood cells to fight the 'invaders'. As a result, the eyes watered, trying to wash away the 'enemy'; the throat tickled to encourage coughing. These unnecessary reactions produced considerable discomfort and congestion, as well as asthma attacks that could become life-threatening. For obvious personal reasons, this new discovery caught my attention.

I've spent the past twenty years studying the immune system. New scientific developments have led me to re-evaluate what I learnt in school – and to pay more attention to the ideas of Ilya Mechnikov. It's now clear that the number one job of the immune system is not to combat germs. Rather, the purpose of the immune system is to allow us to coexist with the microbes in and around us. That means tolerating the harmless ones, as well as fighting those that pose a risk.

SURPRISING CONNECTIONS

Over the past several decades, as it became evident that the incidence of asthma and allergies was rising in the United States, immunologists struggled to find an explanation. One important clue was the fact that these conditions were increasing dramatically in some parts of the world, yet remaining low and stable in others. Statistics suggested a possible connection to antibiotic use. But how were they linked?

A Novel Experiment

In 2002, Dr Mairi Noverr, a postdoctoral research fellow in my laboratory at the University of Michigan Medical Center, was conducting research on the yeast *Candida albicans*. Earlier, while a graduate student in my lab, she had discovered that *C. albicans* released chemicals able to communicate with the immune system. Normally, the population of *C. albicans* in the body is relatively small. But because this yeast is antibiotic-resistant, it proliferates when other microbes are destroyed by antibiotics.

I'd been intrigued by statistical research correlating antibiotics with allergies and asthma. Based on this research and the work we were doing in the lab, I wondered what would happen if we treated mice with antibiotics. This would increase the presence of *C. albicans* and the chemicals it releases, and also reduce the population of probiotics. Perhaps the findings would show a connection between antibiotics and allergies.

Numerous researchers had already worked out ways to develop respiratory allergies in mice. But all of these methods involved either a genetic defect in the mouse or vaccinating the mouse with the allergens. No one had ever got a mouse to develop allergies the way humans do: simply by inhaling an environmental allergen.

Few of my colleagues believed that intestinal microbes could possibly have anything to do with respiratory allergies. But Mairi Noverr was also very intrigued by the idea. We designed and carried out experiments to test it. One group of mice was treated with antibiotics for five days to alter the microbial population of their intestines; the other group received no treatment. All the mice were placed in controlled environments. After they received a course of antibiotics, they were exposed to airborne respiratory allergens for two weeks.

The results were astonishing. The mice that had received antibiotics developed allergies from inhaling the allergens; the others did not. Our experiment confirmed that a microbe in the intestines could affect immune responses elsewhere in the body. After peer review, these exciting findings were published in *Infection and Immunity*, the infection-research journal of the American Society for Microbiology.

Mairi Noverr stayed on in my laboratory as a postdoctoral fellow after she received her PhD, and we continued to collaborate on follow-up studies. She agreed to co-author a chapter of this book that incorporates work we've done together on prebiotics.

The Probiotics Connection

A recent concept in immunology has paved the way for the probiotics revolution: recognising that an immune response, like a car, responds to an accelerator pedal and a brake. Pressing the accelerator launches an immune response, such as inflammation. The response continues until the brake is pressed to stop it. Without the brake to end an inappropriate immune response, the immune system causes disease rather than protecting against it.

We already know, from our experiment and others, that destroying probiotics in the intestines can activate the immune system's accelerator. Preliminary research suggests that probiotics can slam on the brakes.

WHY I WROTE THIS BOOK

We had expected strong interest from scientists when our findings about allergies and antibiotics were announced. But we were caught completely off guard by the outpouring of attention from the media and the public. Stories appeared on Reuters, CBS News, MSNBC, BBC News, in *Forbes* and elsewhere. In interviews, I often mentioned probiotics.

I received heart-rending emails from people who had read these articles and wondered if probiotics could possibly relieve their own terrible medical problem or that of a loved one. Others asked for specific advice on the use of probiotics or shared their personal success with them. I was eager to respond not only to those who contacted me, but to a wider audience of those concerned about the same health issues. But there's another, more personal reason that this topic excites me – one I've rarely shared before now: my own successful use of probiotics.

As a scientist, I'm well aware that one person's experience is hardly proof of a regimen's effectiveness. And I hesitate to sound like an infomercial health guru. But I want you to know that I'm not suggesting that you do anything that I haven't already done myself. In 2002, as my research focused on probiotics, I began to wonder whether they could help me.

At the time, my allergies and asthma had not improved overall since childhood, though the triggers had changed. Summer hay fever was much less of a problem now that I was an adult. But it had been replaced by severe mould allergies. The moulds to which I'm sensitive release their spores at night, so I constantly had a stuffy head in the evening. Since I have the form of asthma that's triggered by allergies, my asthma attacks occurred more frequently at night. During the day, moulds sometimes interfered with my life in other ways. In my part of the United States, many people entertain in basement family rooms – but even finished basements contain mould spores. The pleasure of visiting with friends was often dampened by my allergies. Family camping trips created similar problems.

My doctor had prescribed antihistamines and an inhaler to use as needed. I decided to see if adding probiotics and prebiotics could help. If this additional treatment had involved an unapproved drug, I would have waited for scientific confirmation of its effectiveness and safety. But trying probiotics simply involved healthy dietary changes. How could it hurt to eat yoghurt daily, increase my intake of whole grains, consume more fresh fruit and vegetables, liven up my meals with spices and add a probiotic supplement? Later in the book I'll describe the changes I made and also provide specific instructions about adding probiotics to your diet and using probiotic supplements.

About a month after I started, I was working late on a grant proposal. As usual, there was a box of tissues nearby. When I finished working, I suddenly realised that I hadn't needed to use the tissues, and that I didn't have my usual night-time stuffy nose. Allergies that had been severe for decades had all but disappeared in just a month.

I'm not cured. But respiratory allergies and asthma no longer affect my everyday life. Asthma attacks occur only under exceptional circumstances. For example, I had to use my inhaler when a group of friends and I helped clear out a basement that was extremely wet and mouldy – even my non-allergic friends complained about the air.

Though probiotics research is still in its infancy, I decided it was important to explain the science of probiotics and to provide detailed practical information now, so that health-conscious readers can reap their remarkable benefits. True, we don't yet have all the answers. But probiotics are so safe that there's really no reason to wait.

The book starts with the basics about microbes and the immune system, so you'll understand the role of probiotics in immune system functioning and why microbes in the digestive tract affect the health of every part of the body. In Part 2, I'll discuss specific chronic conditions that probiotics may be able to prevent or treat – including ulcerative colitis and Crohn's disease, allergies, asthma, urinary tract infections, yeast infections, auto-immune diseases, heart disease, obesity and more. By that point, I expect you'll be keen to join the probiotics revolution! Part 3 provides practical information, covering everything you need to know to add probiotics and prebiotics to your life.

We've come a long way in our understanding of microbes since the paper cup generation was in their youth. Modern medicine now appreciates that not all microbes are harmful. Some are our silent partners.

HOW WILL THIS BOOK HELP YOU?

Take this simple quiz to find out – and then check the explanation at the end.

How frequently do you see your GP or healthcare practitioner?

A: Only for medical check-ups.
B: Maybe once or twice a year, when I get ill.
C: Every couple of months for a chronic condition.
D: I'm under medical supervision for a significant health problem.

How often have you taken antibiotics in the past five years?

A: Never.
B: A few times.
C: Once or twice a year.
D: I take antibiotics regularly.

Are you affected by any of the following digestive problems: bloating or gas, acid reflux (heartburn), constipation, diarrhoea, stomach pain?

A: I rarely have any of these difficulties.
B: I experience problems occasionally – for example, when I travel.
C: I often have such symptoms and must be careful about what I eat.
D: Severe digestive difficulties have altered my life.

What happens to you during the cold and flu season?

A: I rarely catch anything, even if I'm looking after someone who's ill.
B: If I stay away from people with symptoms, I'm usually okay.
C: I always get ill once or twice.
D: No matter how careful I am, I come down with whatever is going around.

Do you suffer from respiratory or skin allergies?

A: No.
B: I might have an allergy, but the symptoms are so mild that I'm not sure.
C: I have allergies, but they're not very bad.
D: I have severe allergies.

How often do you get urinary tract or yeast infections?

A: Never.
B: It's happened a couple of times.
C: About once a year.
D: I get them frequently.

Have members of your family been diagnosed with any of the following chronic diseases: inflammatory bowel disease; allergies or asthma; heart disease; autoimmune diseases, such as rheumatoid arthritis, lupus or type 1 diabetes?

A: No.
B: A few relatives in my extended family.
C: One or two members of my immediate family.
D: Both of my parents or more than two members of my immediate family.

Which description best characterises your diet?

A: My diet is excellent, high in whole grains, fruit and vegetables and low in refined carbohydrates and saturated fats.
B: I try to eat healthy foods, but don't always succeed.
C: My diet isn't terrible, but I eat too much junk food.
D: I know I need a complete diet makeover.

Have a look at your answers. Probably the letters are not all the same. But what predominates? If your answers are mostly –

A: Congratulations! Each A answer reflects good health, a robust constitution or health-promoting habits. But even healthy people can benefit from probiotics. Adding probiotics and prebiotics to an already excellent diet makes it even better.
B: These replies suggest that you're already doing pretty well – but certain areas could be improved. Or perhaps you're aware of vulnerabilities and are hoping to stave off problems down the road. The advice in this book could help you make changes to accomplish that goal.
C: Responses in this category suggest that you have health problems or concerns. Though your difficulties aren't life-altering, they're inconvenient. Adding probiotics and prebiotics to your diet, and perhaps also taking an appropriate probiotic supplement, could make a difference. The chapters in this book about relevant conditions will be of particular interest to you.
D: If you answered D to questions about your health, you're coping with significant medical challenges. Probiotics and prebiotics could be an important supplement to the treatments you're already getting. In many cases, they enhance therapeutic benefits or reduce side effects. Because this area of research is expanding so rapidly, even experienced practitioners aren't always aware of all possibilities. The book will provide information that you can discuss with your healthcare provider.

CHAPTER TWO

The Secret World
Within Us

If you could extract all of the trillions of microbes that live in your body, you'd have just under one litre of cream-coloured sludge. But under the microscope, you'd find a fascinating variety of micro-organisms – including probiotics – in a wide variety of shapes and colours. Individual microbes are tiny; few can be seen with the naked eye. But they're hardly a minor component of our body. Together, they weigh more than one kilo. That is more than the kidneys (about 140 grams), pancreas (around 110 grams) and heart (about 230 grams) put together!

The human body consists of about ten trillion cells. In addition, each of us is host to *one hundred trillion* microbes. Thus our microbes outnumber our own cells ten to one. Some scientists joke that we're a minority in our own body. However, rest assured:

on average, human cells are about twenty times as large as a typical microbe. So while we're a minority of cells, we are the majority in terms of sheer bulk (phew!).

Collectively, the microbes we host are known as our microflora. Nearly 80 per cent of them – including all the ones important to the immune system – live in our intestines. The rest reside elsewhere in the digestive tract, on the skin and in the lungs, as well as in the female reproductive tract. If a woman is breastfeeding, the milk-producing areas of her breasts also contain microbes. Other parts of the body, such as the bones, heart, kidneys and other internal organs, are normally microbe-free – unless they're infected.

➤ MICROFLORA VS MICROBIOTA ◄

If you read scientific articles about microbes, you may be puzzled to see the term 'microbiota' used instead of 'microflora'. Technically speaking, 'microbiota' – meaning 'microscopic life' – is correct. So where did 'microflora' come from?

Centuries ago, when microscopes were first developed and the microbes within us were discovered, scientists believed they were a form of plants. The word 'microflora' – literally 'microscopic plants' – was used to describe them. Scientists switched to 'microbiota' once they realised that these tiny life-forms weren't plants after all. But 'microflora' is still the more widely recognised word. So we decided to use this term in the book instead of the scientific one.

We now realise that our microbes are not accidental passengers along for the ride. Collectively, they perform functions essential for our health. In this chapter, I'll introduce the major players and explain what they do. As you'll see, probiotics live in a challenging, competitive environment, so they need our support. Fortunately, we can easily deliver additional probiotics to the gut, simply by swallowing food or supplements that contain them. And we can also boost them with prebiotics, foods that support these beneficial microbes. The goal is to improve immune system functioning and health with a balance of microbes that's optimal for us.

UNDER THE MICROSCOPE

More than 99 per cent of the microbes living in our intestines are bacteria, a very diverse group, with 500 to 1,000 different species. The rest are yeasts or parasites.

Bacteria

We're constantly exposed to staggering numbers of bacteria in the environment, and our own body contains hundreds of types. Many people assume that all bacteria are harmful germs. But, in fact, few bacteria cause disease in humans.

All bacteria are microscopic single-cell life forms. But they're quite diverse in size, as well as shape, colour and growth rate. Bacteria can be shaped like rods, balls, or even spirals. Some are plain, others astonishingly beautiful. Depending on their size, tens of thousands of bacteria – or even hundreds of thousands – could fit on the full stop at the end of this sentence.

Some bacteria, such as *Escherichia coli* (better known as *E. coli*), can double their numbers in as little as twenty minutes. That's why it's so important to refrigerate raw meat, which may contain harmful strains of *E. coli*. If left at room temperature, which is more conducive to their growth, these microbes can rapidly reach levels that cause food poisoning. In contrast, other bacteria, such as *Bacteroides* – the most numerous bacteria in our intestines –

need a few hours to double their population. *Mycobacteria*, the cause of tuberculosis, require almost a day.

➤ UNDERSTANDING MICROBE NAMES ➤

If you look at the label on a bottle of probiotic supplements, you may see something like '*Lactobacillus rhamnosus* GG'. This is what it means:

• The name that appears first, *Lactobacillus* in this case, is the genus — think of it as a clan or extended family name. (By the way, the plural of 'genus' is 'genera'.)

• The name that appears second, *rhamnosus*, designates the particular species within that genus — like a family or surname.

• The name or number that appears third, GG, is the name of the specific strain within that species — like a first name.

You'll probably notice while reading this book that when a microbe is identified in print, the genus and species names (but not the strain name) are italicised, with the genus capitalised. When the microbe is mentioned several times, the genus name is often abbreviated to the first letter, as in *L. rhamnosus* GG.

Bacteria are not only found in people, but in all living creatures — mammals, birds, fish and even insects. Bacteria also live in water and in the earth. Just one teaspoon of rich soil contains over one hundred million bacteria.

You already know that certain bacteria can cause disease in humans. They can cause disease in plants, too. But the great majority of those that live in soil perform positive – and sometimes essential – roles. For example, the friendly bacteria in soil inhibit the growth of bacteria responsible for plant diseases. They also decompose plant matter into simpler molecules that plants can use for food or as nutrients. If you've ever had a working compost pile in your garden, it would have been loaded with helpful bacteria.

Yeasts

Of the remaining microbes in our intestines, nearly all are yeasts – a type of fungus. Each yeast organism consists of a single oval-shaped cell that's larger than a bacterial cell but smaller than a human cell. Like bacteria, yeasts are all around us. They're in the soil and in the air; they live on grains, fruit and vegetables. Centuries ago, yeasts entered the dwellings of our ancestors, found their way into cooking vessels – and brought us the original sourdough bread plus the first fermented beverage to wash it down.

The major yeast of the human microflora is *Candida albicans*. If its numbers are kept low by competition with other microbes, it's harmless. But if it proliferates, it can cause various illnesses, including diarrhoea, vaginal yeast infections and thrush, an infection of the mouth that's common in infants and in people taking antibiotics.

Parasites

Finally, even the healthiest among us are hosts to a few parasites – organisms that depend on us for food and shelter but that offer us nothing in return. At best, they're harmless. But parasites can be a significant cause of disease, especially in the digestive tract. Examples include tapeworms; *Giardia*, a parasite found in lakes and streams that backpackers fear; and *Cryptosporidium*, a parasite that can cause diarrhoea, dehydration, nausea, vomiting and even death. In some parts of the world, such as Africa and South-east Asia, parasite infections are far more common than they are in the United States or Britain. But they can strike here, too. In 1993, *Cryptosporidium* contaminated the water supply of Milwaukee, Wisconsin, in the USA, infecting 403,000 people and causing 69 deaths.

Though I've mentioned parasites to give you an overview of the digestive tract microflora, they won't appear often in this book. That's because parasites are extremely rare in the normal (i.e., uninfected) microflora, and there's no evidence that they play a significant role in health at this extremely low level.

➤ WHAT ABOUT VIRUSES? ➤

Like parasites, viruses may be found in the intestinal tract if we have a viral illness. Some scientists speculate that viruses are part of the normal microflora, in residence whether we're healthy or ill. But we aren't yet certain this is true.

Though both bacteria and viruses are microbes, their structures are quite different. Bacteria are independent one-celled organisms. Viruses are like capsules filled with genes. They don't live independently; rather, they invade other cells and take them over. When the invaded cells reproduce, the new cells also contain the virus. If the virus can cause disease, the disease spreads.

Because of these structural characteristics, antibiotics can't kill viruses or the cells that contain them. That's why doctors try to ascertain that an illness is bacterial rather than viral in origin before prescribing antibiotics to treat it.

OUR COMPLEX RELATIONSHIPS WITH THE MICROBES WITHIN US

In exchange for our hospitality, our microflora supplies services important for health. Some microbes are purely beneficial. Others are never helpful and can cause disease if their numbers rise too high. But a much larger number of microbes are sometimes good and sometimes bad for our health, depending on their population size and location.

Probiotic Microbes

Healthy people have high levels of probiotic bacteria – and the more, the better. Probiotics protect us by competing with harmful microbes and by helping the immune system to function. Of the most numerous probiotics in our microflora, the two we know the most about are:

- *Lactobacillus*, the bacteria found in fermented dairy products, such as yoghurt
- *Bifidobacterium*, also found in some yoghurts

We host many species of *Lactobacillus* and *Bifidobacterium*. Some probiotics aren't considered part of the microflora, because they're not normally in residence. But if they happen to pass through the digestive tract, they're able to exert positive effects on health. These transient microbes include some species of *Lactobacillus*, as well as some soil microbes, believe it or not. Note: I'm *not* suggesting that you add soil to your diet! Some soil microbes are dangerous.

Harmful Microbes

Other microbes – fortunately a small minority – are the 'bad guys' of the microflora. We can't avoid them completely. If their population is kept in check by other microbes, they aren't dangerous. But if their numbers increase too much, they can cause disease and may affect how well the immune system functions. As far as we know at the moment, they offer no benefits. Some common examples are:

- *Candida albicans*, the yeast that causes yeast infections
- *Clostridium difficile*, a bacterium that causes diarrhoea
- *Pseudomonas aeruginosa*, a bacterium that causes pneumonia

Microbes That Can Help or Harm

At low levels, certain potentially harmful bacteria actually contribute to good health. But if they're allowed to proliferate – or if they migrate from the intestines to other places in the body – they could cause problems. Two examples are:

- *Bacteroides* are the most numerous bacteria in the intestines of healthy individuals. They contribute to intestinal tract health and may help to digest dietary carbohydrates. However, if certain strains of *Bacteroides* move beyond the intestines, they can cause bacterial abscesses.
- *Klebsiella* are helpful at low levels – they make vitamins B_{12} and K. But if they're allowed to grow too much, or if they migrate from the intestines to other places in the body, they can become harmful. For example, *Klebsiella* infection of the lungs is one of the leading causes of bacterial pneumonia.

INSIDE OUR OUTSIDE

The inside of your body consists of all the areas where your blood vessels and internal organs lie: the liver, kidneys, brain, heart, etc. Your insides are essentially microbe-free – at least when you're healthy.

The body's outside includes the skin. But you might be surprised to learn that it also includes the lungs and upper airways, plus the 'tube' that runs right through the middle of us. This tube consists of the nose, sinuses, upper airways, lungs, mouth, oesophagus, stomach, small and large intestines, rectum, and anus. They're considered 'outside' because they're constantly exposed to the world around us. This exposure allows microbes to enter our body via the food we eat, the fluids we drink and the air we inhale. Some of these microbes take up residence in the tube – the vast majority of them in the gut – and become part of our microflora.

Protecting the Tube

Exposure to the outside world makes the tube vulnerable, but its surface has an important protective mechanism: mucus. The lining of the tube is made of mucosal (i.e., mucus-producing) surfaces. Even when you don't have a cold, mucus coats all the mucosal surfaces. When a microbe from the outside world lands in the tube, the immune system registers it as friend or foe. If it's a friend, the immune system tolerates its presence. The mucosal surfaces actually feed microbes categorised as friendly. One reason that mucus is sticky is that it contains sugar, which microbes use as food.

Foes, on the other hand, are trapped by mucus and expelled from the body. If this mucus is in the respiratory tract, it may exit via the nose or mouth. But most of it is carried out through the digestive tract. Cilia – tiny hair-like projections from cells in the airways – serve as brooms, sweeping microbe-laden mucus into the mouth. Without always being aware of it, we automatically swallow many times an hour. This pushes not only excess saliva, but also mucus and microbes, down the tube. Next, peristalsis – the rhythmic muscular squeezing of the digestive tract – takes over. Swallowed material moves from the throat to the stomach, through the intestines and rectum, to the anus, which expels it from the body.

➤ 'EVERYTHING WE INHALE, WE ALSO SWALLOW' ◄

Our laboratory at the University of Michigan introduced this intriguing concept to help explain how the intestinal tract can affect immune responses in the respiratory tract. It's easy to understand that everything we eat or drink ends up in the intestines. But what about allergens and other particles in the air we breathe?

During allergy season we inhale approximately one thousand pollen spores every hour. But it's a tortuous path from nose or mouth to the lungs. More than half of the pollen spores we inhale never complete the journey. Instead, they get stuck in the mucus of the sinuses, mouth, throat and upper airways. This mucus is swallowed – and it ends up in the gut. Thanks to the mucosa, our intestinal tract is exposed to everything we inhale.

A Competitive Environment

The tube within us is teeming with microbes, all competing to survive. Our microfloral balance – and thus our health – depends on which ones succeed. Microbes compete with each other in several ways:

- **Use of nutrients:** Competition favours microbes that can make use of available nutrients. We can give probiotic bacteria the edge with a diet high in fibre, a prebiotic, because probiotics can digest fibre, whereas many harmful bacteria cannot. On the other hand, sugary foods help certain harmful microbes to thrive.

Our Internal Tube

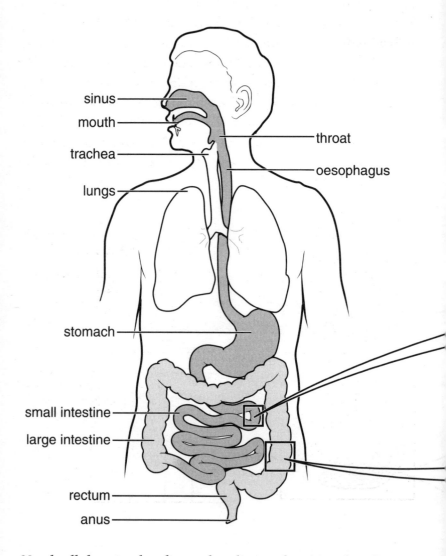

Nearly all the microbes that we host live on the mucosal surfaces that line the tube running through the centre of our body.

• **Access to intestinal cells:** A microbe can survive longer in the gut if it can stick to cells of the intestines. Otherwise, it's likely to be swept out of the body by peristalsis. One of the ways probiotic bacteria help to protect us from harmful microbes is by successfully competing with them for access to intestinal cells.

• **Production of antimicrobial chemicals:** Some bacteria produce their own antibiotics. These chemicals don't affect us, but they inhibit the growth of other bacteria. Also, as microbes digest food, their metabolic by-products may have adverse effects on their competitors. For example, when probiotics use fibre as their nutritional source, some of their metabolic by-products are acids similar to vinegar – and yeasts don't grow well in the presence of these acids.

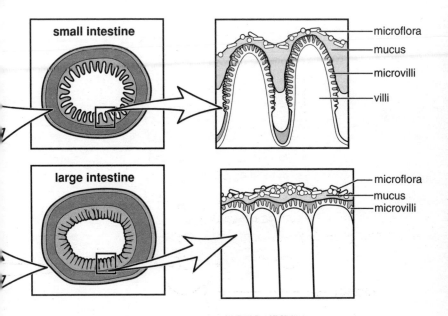

Our Microbial Neighbourhoods

The microbial population of our digestive tract varies from place to place along the tube. Different types of microbes predominate at each site, and they serve different functions. In the upper part of the digestive tract, probiotics mainly compete with harmful microbes; the same is true of the lower end. This means that their impact is local. Probiotics in the intestines, which can actually affect the immune system, are the most important for overall well-being.

Mouth

The balance of microbes in our mouth helps determine our oral health. Probiotics counter cavities by keeping *Streptococcus mutans* under control; these are the bacteria that can cause tooth decay if their numbers are high enough. Other bacteria, such as *Porphyromonas gingivalis*, may lead to gum disease if not kept in check by competing microbes.

Stomach

The stomach produces acid so strong that it could burn a hole in your living room carpet. Though many microbes can survive the passage through the stomach, few are able to live there. The most notable of these is the bacterium *Helicobacter pylori*, which is responsible for ulcers. *H. pylori* produces chemicals that neutralise acid in their vicinity, allowing them to survive. Certain probiotics – including species of *Lactobacillus* – can also live in the stomach. They help to prevent ulcers by keeping *H. pylori* numbers low.

Small and Large Intestines

Food travels from the stomach to the small intestine, where it's broken down into components our body can use for fuel. Most of our nutrient absorption occurs in the small intestine. In the large intestine, more nutrients and water are extracted.

The large majority of the microbes in our microflora live in the intestines. This is also where the most important communication between microbes and the immune system occurs, as I'll describe in Chapter 4. The intestines are particularly well suited for microbial growth and colonisation. That's because they're over nine metres long and their surface consists of numerous tiny folds – called villi and microvilli – in which microbes can live. The villi and microvilli serve as more than residence for microbes. They also help us to absorb nutrients because of the huge surface area they provide. In fact, if you could uncoil and unfold the intestines, the flattened tissue would be larger than a tennis court!

The bacterial population of the large intestine outnumbers that of the small intestine by about 100,000 to 1. That's because the small intestine is less hospitable to microbes: its environment is more acidic and has a higher concentration of both digestive enzymes and antimicrobial chemicals. In addition, peristalsis is significantly faster in the small intestine.

As you might guess from the environmental differences, different types of bacteria normally live in the small and large intestines. The predominant bacteria in the small intestine are benign species of *Streptococcus* and *Enterococcus.* Though they are important in maintaining a healthy microflora balance, like many microbes in the gut, they can cause disease if found in high enough numbers in another location. In the large intestine, *Bacteroides* dominates. Probiotics can be found all along the small and large intestines. Their presence is a major force in maintaining a healthy balance among the intestinal microbes.

Rectum and Anus

The rectum collects wastes and expels them through the anus in the form of faeces. Microbes don't actually live in the rectum or anus. However, they pass through in huge numbers. One-third of our faeces consist of bacteria. Though most of these are harmless, some can make you ill. That's why it's vitally important to take measures, from sewage treatment to hand-washing, to prevent dangerous expelled microbes from re-entering the mouth.

THE BALANCING ACT

The process of maintaining a balanced microflora is similar in complexity – and mystery – to maintaining our weight. Few of us follow exactly the same dietary and exercise regimen every day. On a busy day we may move more and eat less; at the weekend we may sit about and eat more. But our weight doesn't vary nearly as much as these differences might suggest. It takes significant and persistent changes – switching from a sedentary job to an active one; making a habit of fast-food meals – to produce lasting losses or gains.

The same is true of our microflora balance. Our gut microflora consists of many types of microbes, and new ones constantly enter the tube. Everything we inhale, eat, drink or touch is a source of microbes; we also pick them up in our interactions with other people and with animals. Nevertheless, each of us somehow reaches a balance that remains remarkably consistent – provided we don't disrupt it. But unfortunately, most of us have unknowingly done just that.

During the past forty to fifty years, many of us have inadvertently performed a massive experiment by making two significant lifestyle modifications: greatly increasing our use of antibiotics and substantially changing our diet. Together, these changes have produced an invisible epidemic of insufficient probiotics. As a result, the balance of our intestinal microbe population has changed, sometimes with disastrous effects on our immune system – and major consequences for public health.

Exposure to Antibiotics

Antibiotics have the most profound impact on a person's microflora. Their use in healthcare and in agriculture has increased dramatically since penicillin became widely available at the end of the Second World War. Though these drugs are an essential weapon against dangerous microbes, they kill the beneficial ones, too. A typical two-week course of high-dose antibiotic treatment, as might be used for an ear infection, can wipe out most of the normal gut microbes.

After treatment, the microflora grows back. But probiotic bacteria recover more slowly than other microbes, particularly if a person's diet is high in refined carbohydrates and low in prebiotics. Unless the problem is corrected, the microbial balance after taking antibiotics will be different from what it was before, with likely lingering ill effects to the immune system. Later in the book I'll describe the often neglected second part of antibiotic treatment: measures to restore microbial balance.

In addition to occasional medicinal doses of antibiotics, we're exposed to them at the much lower levels sometimes found in meats and drinking water. But these doses may be frequent rather than occasional. Such exposure can produce subtle long-term changes in our microflora. As this book will explain, we can counter the problem by increasing our intake of foods that contain probiotics or that foster their growth.

The New Diet

Whatever we eat, our gut microbes eat. But different types of microbes have different food preferences. Depending on what we consume, some microbes will thrive while others go hungry. Thus our diet is a major factor in regulating the balance among the various microbes in our microflora.

The current diet of most industrialised nations has changed dramatically in recent decades. We now consume one out of every three meals away from home, and even those meals eaten at home are often prepared elsewhere. The result is a diet with more highly processed ingredients, less fresh fruit and vegetables, less whole grains and less fibre. At the same time, many people are eating more sugar and more fat, particularly more fat of animal origin.

You've heard this list of dietary changes before, because they've caused obesity rates to soar. Less well known is the fact that each of these changes can also favour the growth of potentially harmful microbes over probiotics. Laboratory studies have compared the microflora of rats fed a healthy diet (high in fibre and low in fat and table sugar) with the microflora of rats whose diet is the opposite – low in fibre and high in fat and table sugar. The two groups of rats have significantly different bacterial populations growing in their intestinal tracts. In addition, the bacteria associated with a healthy diet are better able to break down carcinogens in food – a connection I'll explore further in Chapter 9. Animal studies also show that simple carbohydrates can increase the growth of *Candida albicans* in the intestines.

✺ IS THERE A GENETICALLY DETERMINED ✺ MICROFLORA 'FINGERPRINT'?

Some studies suggest that each of us has a unique microflora, a kind of fingerprint of the major types of microbes in our gut. Moreover, investigators have shown that the microfloras of identical twins are more similar than those of fraternal twins, which are, in turn, more similar than those of two unrelated individuals. These findings suggest that our microflora is at least partly determined by our genes. However, environmental factors – particularly antibiotic use and diet – have the strongest influence on the make-up of the microflora.

In Search of the Optimal Balance

The challenge to medical researchers is how best to define a microflora balance that promotes health. We have rough guidelines that are comparable to the old height-weight tables found on the scales in chemists. But as with weight, what's healthy varies from individual to individual.

For example, studies of the microflora of healthy people have found that *Bacteroides* is the most numerous bacterium in the gut. It typically outnumbers *E. coli* by over one thousand to one and outnumbers *Candida* by over one million to one. However, this is like saying that people should consume 2,000 calories per day on average. True – but this average doesn't apply to everyone, male or female, young or old, sedentary or active. Similarly, some people can remain healthy with relatively low levels of probiotics, while others require much higher levels.

At the moment, the best way to determine if your microflora is balanced is to consider your overall state of health. If you're fortunate enough to feel healthy, energetic and in good spirits – and if you normally resist contagious illnesses (and bounce back quickly on the rare occasions when you do succumb) – chances are that your microflora and immune system are in excellent shape.

SHOULD YOU TAKE A TEST TO ANALYSE YOUR GUT MICROFLORA?

Many companies offer tests that claim to analyse your gut microflora. You can find a laboratory online or in an advertisement in a health-related publication. After you pay for the test (typically a few hundred pounds), you follow instructions for obtaining a stool sample, and post it. The company will culture the sample in their laboratory and then examine the culture under a microscope. The report they return usually includes an analysis of the types of bacteria and yeasts the sample contained, plus warnings about problems, such as parasites and imbalances.

These tests can be helpful in some cases – for example, if the numbers are extremely abnormal. Some practitioners have extensive experience with them and can offer anecdotal evidence of their benefits. But this isn't something that's been confirmed by peer-reviewed research.

I wish I could give you clear guidance about these tests, but I can't. On one hand, I'm reluctant to dismiss the opinion of the experienced healthcare providers who use them. But on the other, I want to offer a few caveats.

It's important to understand that stool tests of this nature cannot provide a complete overview of your microflora. Many of our gut microbes require complex procedures to be cultured successfully – and some can't be grown outside the body at all. Moreover, there's currently no consensus in the medical community about how to interpret the results of these tests. I look forward to more research in this area, both to develop more comprehensive tests and also to learn how to use them to design effective therapies.

On the other hand, if you suffer from chronic medical problems, there could be a gut-microbe connection. Despite the body's intricate mechanisms for maintaining a healthy microflora, the balance of microbes can be toppled by other forces. Changes in this balance can lead to chronic health problems. Our best defence against this is to provide the corrective force of probiotics and prebiotics in our diet.

CHAPTER THREE

Antibiotics: A Medical Miracle with a Dark Side

I know about the lifesaving power of antibiotics first-hand. When my daughter was five, she pricked her left hand on a rosebush thorn in our garden. The problem didn't seem serious at first. But the next day she had a fever. In her left armpit was a lymph node so enlarged that it looked like a golf ball under her skin. A puzzling red streak ran from her left wrist halfway up her arm.

Doctors diagnosed an acute bacterial infection. Half a century ago, a child might have died from such an infection. But my daughter received antibiotics. After a day of intravenous treatment, she was better. To ensure that the infection was completely eliminated, she remained on antibiotic tablets for two weeks.

Antibiotics are true miracle drugs. Penicillin was developed first, just in time to treat soldiers during the Second World War.

Late in the war, it became available to civilians. Other antibiotics soon followed. By 1950, antibiotic treatment had become a routine part of medical care. The impact on public health was extraordinary. Deaths due to bacterial diseases and infections plummeted. Yet we're now learning that this miracle has a dark side, because of how we have used and abused antibiotics over the last fifty years.

ANTIBIOTIC GLOSSARY

The word 'antibiotic' comes from the Greek *anti*, meaning 'against', and *bios*, meaning 'life'.

Antibiotics are chemical compounds that are themselves derived from microbes. They can kill bacteria, but they don't affect other microbes, such as viruses and yeasts.

Antibacterial compounds also kill bacteria, but this term is generally reserved for synthetic compounds rather than ones made from microbes.

Antimicrobials are compounds that kill not only bacteria but also other forms of microbes.

THE DISCOVERY OF PENICILLIN

The story of how penicillin was developed fascinates me, because it features the finest elements of breakthrough scientific research: perseverance, intuition, creativity – and luck. Penicillin was discovered in 1928 by Dr Alexander Fleming, a British physician and researcher who was known for being bright but untidy. At the time, he was studying *Staphylococcus*, bacteria that can cause food poisoning and infections. He returned from his summer holiday to find neglected cultures that were contaminated by mould. But as he examined the ruined dishes of *Staphylococcus*, he noticed something unexpected: in the areas near the mould, bacterial growth was inhibited.

The mould turned out to be a type of *Penicillium*, one of the moulds that grow on bread and other foods. Fleming developed an extract of the mould and named it 'penicillin'. Over the next few years, he conducted a series of experiments with it. He learnt that his penicillin extract could inhibit some harmful bacteria. Moreover, when he injected it into laboratory animals, it caused no harmful symptoms.

Though Fleming published these promising initial findings, he couldn't produce enough penicillin to go further. Doubting that his discovery had any practical value, he turned his attention elsewhere. But several years later, two Oxford University scientists – Howard Florey and Ernest Chain – took up the investigation.

In 1940, Florey and Chain injected eight mice with a dose of *Streptococcus* bacteria that was sufficient to cause a lethal infection. An hour later, they injected four of the mice with penicillin; the others were left untreated. The results were dramatic: the next day, all of the untreated mice were dead, but all that had received penicillin were alive.

Florey and Chain were eager to try penicillin on humans. But people are about three thousand times larger than mice; consequently, their treatment requires much larger quantities of a drug. Months of labour were required to produce enough penicillin for just two patients. The first was a police constable who – like my daughter many years later – had scratched himself on a rosebush. The scratch, which was on his face, had become infected, and the infection had spread to his eyes, scalp, arms and lungs. By the time he was injected with penicillin, he was near death. After only one day in which he received injections every three hours, the constable's condition had improved remarkably; four days later, he seemed almost cured. Since doctors expected him to recover fully, they used all the remaining penicillin to treat a second patient.

That patient survived, but the constable suffered a relapse. Additional penicillin probably would have saved him, but there was none. Tragically, he died from his infection.

Clearly, the potential of penicillin was enormous. But it could not be realised until large-scale production methods were developed. The Second World War had begun, and Britain's research resources were limited. So Florey and Chain turned to the US government. In previous wars, more soldiers had died from disease and infections than from bullets and other weapons. Thus penicillin had tremendous potential to save soldiers' lives and strengthen the war effort. In 1943, the US War Production Board – established to maximise production of essential products – took over responsibility for manufacturing penicillin. Thanks to a massive effort involving leading drug manufacturers, penicillin production soared and countless lives were saved on the battlefield. In 1945, Fleming, Florey and Chain shared the Nobel Prize in Medicine for the discovery of penicillin.

By the time the war ended, penicillin production was sufficient for civilian use. The new drug became available in every chemist in America and Britain. Many other antibiotics followed, starting with streptomycin. Moreover, the use of antibiotics quickly expanded beyond injections and tablets for ill people.

You're undoubtedly aware that many products found in your local chemists and shops contain small doses of antibiotics or antibacterials: topical antibiotic creams to apply to small wounds, as well as antibacterial soaps, washing-up liquids, sponges, dish-cloths and chopping boards. Less visible, but far more significant, are agricultural applications. In 2000, the Centers for Disease Control and Prevention (CDC) and the Animal Health Institute estimated that 20 million kilos of antibiotics were produced annually in the United States. Of that amount, 18 million pounds – 36 per cent – were used in agriculture. Similar agricultural practices were being followed in the UK at that time.

We take antibiotics for granted now. If you were born after the

Second World War, it may be difficult to appreciate how these drugs transformed public health. Life-threatening diseases – such as bacterial pneumonia, scarlet fever and dysentery – suddenly could be vanquished in days. Antibiotics reduced or eliminated infectious complications from traumatic injuries and burns. Infections from childbirth and surgery were readily treated. And a ruptured appendix was no longer the death sentence it had been for my uncle Jimmy. By the 1960s, these stunning successes led the medical community to believe that the war against microbes and infectious disease had been won. As the use of antibiotics spread, no one knew that new epidemics were about to begin.

HOW ANTIBIOTICS WORK

When we take an antibiotic, we hope it will kill the particular bacterium that's making us ill. But antibiotics don't work with surgical precision. All of them affect many bacteria in our micro-flora, including beneficial ones. Some of the consequences are obvious – just read the list of side effects on the package insert. But other effects are more subtle and less well known. Happily, we're learning that probiotics can prevent or correct many of these problems.

A Spectrum of Effectiveness

Antibiotics kill bacteria in different ways. For instance, penicillin disrupts the building of cell walls in certain bacteria. The cell wall, a very strong coating that surrounds each bacterium, protects it from salts and other potentially harmful chemicals. Without an intact cell wall, bacteria break open and die. Another example: tetracycline interferes with the ability of particular bacteria to produce proteins they need to grow. Other antibiotics work via different mechanisms.

Each antibiotic affects some bacteria but not others. The penicillin originally isolated by Alexander Fleming was highly effective against *Staphylococcus* and certain other bacteria, but not against *E. coli*. However, different antibiotics can counter *E. coli*. The list of bacteria vulnerable to a particular antibiotic is referred to as its 'spectrum of activity'. A broad-spectrum antibiotic kills many different kinds of bacteria. However, no antibiotic has been discovered that's effective against all of them.

Side Effects

When you take an antibiotic, some bacteria – plus all yeasts – are left unharmed. With their competition out of the way, they thrive. This selective slaughter changes the microflora balance, explaining such common side effects of antibiotics as the following:

• Diarrhoea, due to overgrowth of *Clostridia diffioilo*, which resists most antibiotics
• Vaginal yeast infections in women, caused by *Candida*, whose proliferation is normally prevented by *Lactobacillus*, a probiotic that's vulnerable to many antibiotics
• Oral thrush, a disease caused when *Candida* infects the mucous membranes of the mouth. *Candida* growth is normally controlled in the mouth by a combination of oral bacteria and the immune system. If antibiotic treatment destroys the oral bacteria, the immune system alone cannot control growth of this yeast.

The Hidden Consequences of Antibiotic Treatment

Within a week after antibiotic treatment ends, the microflora partly recovers its normal balance. In most cases, the side effects go away. What's not obvious, though, is that the microflora balance remains disrupted.

As I mentioned in Chapter 2, our genetic programming appears to dictate the balances among some of the major types of bacteria that live within us. These will quickly be restored to what they were before antibiotics. In contrast, a return to pre-antibiotic levels is more difficult for bacteria that are usually less numerous in our microflora.

Some types of bacteria will be partly or completely wiped out by a course of antibiotics. Over time, they'll be re-introduced into our bodies as we breathe, eat, drink and otherwise expose ourselves to the world. However, the decimated populations may be slow to return to their previous levels, because the bacteria are now relatively few in number and must compete for nutrients with other bacteria that survived antibiotic treatment more successfully. The microflora balance is also affected by proliferation of bacteria and yeasts that weren't affected by the antibiotic. Their higher-than-normal populations usually diminish slowly as their natural competitors recover, though their numbers may remain elevated.

Probiotics are easily killed by antibiotics, and their recovery is quite variable. As a result, the post-antibiotic microflora is likely to be deficient in probiotics. But we can do a lot to correct this. The single greatest influence on probiotic recovery is diet. That's why eating foods that contain probiotics is important both during and after antibiotic treatment: this keeps their numbers high. Recovery is also boosted by consuming foods high in prebiotics, compounds that promote probiotic growth. Conversely, a poor diet – such as one high in sugar – can impede restoration of probiotics in the gut. Adding probiotic supplements is another way to promote a speedy return to healthy levels. In Chapter 11, I'll provide specific recommendations for aiding microflora recovery after antibiotic treatment.

BACTERIA FIGHT BACK

Antibiotics are remarkably powerful weapons. But bacteria are a wily enemy – one that can evolve to protect itself. This phenomenon is called antibiotic resistance: the ability of normally susceptible bacteria to become impervious to an antibiotic. When that happens, a highly effective medication suddenly ceases to work. Decades of medical progress are wiped out, and, once again, we're vulnerable to a bacterial infection.

Every time an antibiotic is prescribed, there's a risk of creating new resistant strains. As I'll explain in Part 2, medical researchers are exploring ways to use probiotics instead of antibiotics to prevent or treat certain conditions. The hope is that probiotics could reduce levels of certain harmful bacteria through a natural process of competition. This approach would not only reduce side effects, but also the risk of antibiotic resistance.

How Resistance Develops

At his Nobel Lecture in 1945, Fleming sounded an alarm about antibiotic resistance. Here's how he explained it:

> *The time may come when penicillin can be bought by anyone in the shops. Then there is the danger that the ignorant man may easily underdose himself and by exposing his microbes to non-lethal quantities of the drug make them resistant. Here is a hypothetical illustration. Mr X has a sore throat. He buys some penicillin and gives himself not enough to kill the Streptococci but enough to educate them to resist penicillin. He then infects his wife. Mrs X gets pneumonia and is treated with penicillin. As the Streptococci are now resistant to penicillin, the treatment fails. Mrs X dies. Who is primarily responsible for Mrs X's death? Why, Mr X whose negligent use of penicillin changed the nature of the microbe.*

If antibiotic doses aren't strong enough to eliminate the infection-causing bacteria completely, the bacteria have the opportunity to mutate. Some of the mutants may survive, despite the antibiotic. As exposure to insufficient doses continues, these resistant strains proliferate while the original strain continues to succumb. If a person becomes infected with the mutant strain, the antibiotic is useless.

With few exceptions, we've managed to stay ahead of resistant bacteria by developing new antibiotics or modifying old ones. Despite these efforts, the prevalence of antibiotic resistance continues to increase. Experts are concerned about one especially frightening possibility: the rise of 'superbugs' – bacteria that can cause serious disease and that are resistant to all available antibiotics.

A New Problem: Chronic Low-Level Exposure to Antibiotics

We're exposed to antibiotics, even if we never take them for an illness. As I mentioned earlier in the chapter, they're used extensively in agriculture. Sometimes the purpose is to treat infections in livestock. But far more significant is the routine practice of giving small daily doses to uninfected animals in their feed.

Low doses of antibiotics improve the general health of livestock, increase reproduction and reduce the death rate. However, the major benefit is an economic one: antibiotics increase feed efficiency – how much weight animals gain for each kilo of feed they consume. Adding antibiotics can increase the weight of an animal by 15 per cent. For example, a pig that would normally reach 90 kilos on a given amount of feed gains 13 extra kilos without consuming any more. While it's economically advantageous to increase feed efficiency in livestock, there are also disturbing drawbacks to using antibiotics in this way.

SIMPLE MEASURES TO PREVENT ANTIBIOTIC RESISTANCE

To prevent antibiotic resistance, it's important only to use these powerful drugs when necessary – and to use them wisely.

• **Take antibiotics only when appropriate.** Sometimes patients demand antibiotic prescriptions when they're not indicated, as for the common cold, which is viral in origin. And the problem isn't limited to patients. Before the risk of resistance became widely known, some doctors prescribed antibiotics for illnesses caused by viruses or yeasts, even though these non-bacterial microbes aren't killed by antibiotics. But this has changed. According to a study published in the *Journal of the American Medical Association*, surgery-based doctors wrote 40 per cent fewer prescriptions for antibiotics for children and adolescents in 1999 to 2000 than they had ten years earlier.

• **Complete antibiotic treatment, even if symptoms are gone.** Resistance can occur when antibiotics are not kept at high enough levels in the body for a sufficiently long time. That's why doctors prescribe treatment over a period of days. Unfortunately, some people stop taking antibiotics as soon as their symptoms disappear. But an apparent return to health doesn't mean that the disease-causing bacteria have been eradicated.

In 2001, a study appeared in the *New England Journal of Medicine* reporting that antibiotic-resistant bacteria had been found in supermarket samples of ground chicken, beef, turkey and pork.

Two additional studies in the same issue of the journal reported on the isolation of antibiotic-resistant bacteria in chicken and pork. Meanwhile, European scientists were finding high levels of antibiotics in streams and drinking water. They traced this discovery to the routine use of antibiotics in agriculture.

➤➤ AN ALARMING SCIENCE FAIR PROJECT ➤➤

In 1999, Ashley Mulroy, a high school student in West Virginia, USA, undertook an ambitious science fair project. She had read about European studies reporting antibiotics in streams and drinking water, and decided to see if the same was true in her own town. For her project, she took water samples from the Ohio River, near the town of Wheeling, as well as from local drinking water. The samples were tested for three antibiotics: penicillin, tetracycline and vancomycin.

American scientists had been concerned that low levels of antibiotics in the water supply could promote antibiotic resistance. But Ashley's research drew national attention to the issue. She discovered trace amounts of all three antibiotics in both river water and drinking water samples.

These and other findings have prompted leading infectious disease specialists to urge a ban on routine use of low-dose antibiotics simply to aid animal growth. They argue that public health could be compromised if the practice leads to new disease-causing bacteria that no existing antibiotic can treat.

Sweden adopted such a ban in 1986; Denmark followed in 2000. As concern escalated, so did corrective measures. The entire European Union agreed to ban the routine use of antibiotics in animal feed, starting in 2006. Individual companies have cut or eliminated the use of antibiotics to promote animal growth. For example, in 2005, McDonald's announced that their poultry suppliers worldwide could no longer promote growth with antibiotics used in human medicine. Several leading American chicken suppliers have almost completely ended antibiotic use. And the US Food and Drug Administration is considering new regulations to reduce antibiotic use in livestock feed.

⋙ PLAIN SOAP AND WATER IS STILL THE BEST ⋘

In 2005, Allison Aiello, an assistant professor of epidemiology at the University of Michigan, testified before the FDA's Non-Prescription Drug Advisory Committee on the possibility that triclosan, an anti-bacterial agent found in anti-bacterial soaps, could lead to antibiotic resistance. An increasing number of liquid soaps and other products – including toothpaste – include triclosan as an ingredient.

Dr Aiello's message for the public: though washing hands with soap and water is important for preventing disease transmission, it's not necessary to use anti-bacterial soaps. Research shows that they aren't any more effective than plain soap at removing bacteria from the skin. And they could contribute to antibiotic resistance.

NEW EPIDEMICS

Epidemiologists tracking health trends proclaimed the triumph of antibiotics as deaths from infectious disease fell in the 1950s and 1960s. But by the mid-1990s, they had confirmed a rise in two chronic conditions: allergies and asthma. According to a landmark Center for Disease Control study, asthma rates in the United States increased over 80 per cent from 1980 to 1995; the largest increase was reported for children aged 0 to 4 – a whopping 160 per cent. Subsequent reports up to 2003 on childhood asthma rates continue to show these high levels. The asthma problem is not limited to the United States. The United Kingdom currently has the highest worldwide asthma rate, with over 10 million adults affected.

As these new epidemics revealed themselves, the National Institutes of Health launched a research effort to understand their underlying causes. Several epidemiological studies identified a correlation between early antibiotic use in children and the later development of allergies and asthma. Subsequent research found a link between multiple ear infections early in childhood, a problem usually treated with multiple courses of antibiotics, and the later development of asthma. I'll describe the research linking antibiotic use and allergies in more detail in Chapter 7.

We've only recently begun to appreciate the unfortunate role of antibiotics in chronic diseases that originate in the immune system. So far, most research has focused on asthma and allergies. But antibiotic connections are under investigation for many other conditions, from inflammatory bowel disease to autoimmunity to autism.

Antibiotics are indeed wonder drugs – essential to combat disease. But like any other medication, they have unintended side effects. Some of these side effects are temporary and relatively minor (for example, yeast infections); others last longer and are of greater concern, such as diarrhoea due to *Clostridium difficile* overgrowth. But most significant of all are effects on the immune system, which are far more serious and may last for a lifetime. That's why we must heed the warnings to use these potent drugs more carefully. Fortunately, we're discovering that most, if not all, antibiotic side effects can be prevented by consuming probiotics and prebiotics both during and after treatment.

CHAPTER FOUR

The Immune System, Inflammation and the Gut

We live in a dirty, dangerous world. Every time we breathe, eat, drink, touch or share a kiss, we're exposed to microbes that produce poisons and destructive chemicals. Protecting us from harm is our personal security force: the immune system. Thanks to our immune system, nearly all of us can enjoy kissing and remain healthy, too.

Graduate students in my department take courses in immunology that occupy up to nine hours per week for an entire academic year. They need all that time to learn about the immune system because it's amazingly complicated. And there's still so much we don't know. That's what makes immunology such a fascinating field. To cram the basics into one brief chapter, I'll need to simplify a lot. But I want you to understand some of the most exciting recent developments in immunology – including new recognition that inflammation plays a key role in our health. All of this explains why probiotics hold so much promise for preventing and curing many chronic diseases.

THE BASICS

Our body is a giant community: our own cells, the trillions of microbes we host and many trillions of molecules from the outside world that are just passing through. The immune system is on alert 24/7, maintaining law and order in this complex, varied population. I'll start with a quick overview of how things work, and then give you two examples that show the immune system in action.

Keeping Watch

In contrast to other systems of the body, like the respiratory or digestive system, the immune system isn't stuck in one place. Instead of having organs like the lungs or stomach, the immune system consists of white blood cells. These circulate throughout the body like a mobile police force. White blood cells travel on two pathways: the blood vessels and the similar network of lymphatic vessels (see the box on the next page). But these cells also can exit the pathway, literally squeezing out of the vessels and crawling through our tissues.

Every tissue and organ in our body contains white blood cells, which monitor the microbes inside us. They keep a particularly close watch on the intestines, because that's where the action is. Everything we eat or drink ends up in the gut. Remember the mucus-lined 'tube' I described in Chapter 2, which runs through our centre? All the microbes that live in the upper part – in our sinuses, mouth, airways, throat, oesophagus, and stomach – eventually die and are carried by mucus through the intestinal tract. The same is true for particles we inhale. They get stuck in the mucus of the nose, mouth or airways and get swept down into the gut. By putting the spotlight on the intestines, the immune system can scrutinise most of the microbes in the body, as well as everything we inhale or consume.

➤ LYMPH ➤

Lymph is a clear liquid, rich in white blood cells. It flows through us via lymphatic vessels, which are intertwined with our blood vessels. Along the lymphatic pathway are the equivalents of rest stops: our lymph nodes. Each of us has hundreds of these nodes throughout our body, but they're clustered in certain areas, such as the neck and armpits.

When white blood cells gather in large numbers to stage an attack on harmful microbes, they crowd into the lymph nodes. That's why swollen lymph nodes can be a sign of infection. If your doctor checks your neck and underarms during an examination, it's probably to see if your lymph nodes are enlarged.

Meet the Security Force

Our immune system consists of more than two dozen different types of white blood cells, all produced in our bone marrow. Each has particular jobs to do. To keep things simple, I'll discuss only the most relevant ones.

Lymphocytes (Officers)

Lymphocytes are the brains of the immune system. Depending upon how you characterise them, there are at least eight kinds of lymphocytes, which perform different tasks as they patrol our body. But we'll focus on just three. Two types are called T cells because they go through quality control in the thymus, a small gland tucked between the breastbone and the heart. The other type is called B cells, because their quality control takes place in the bone marrow.

• **Helper T cells** are detective lymphocytes. Each specialises in a particular harmful molecule, much like a detective with expertise in counterfeiters, drug-dealers or serial killers. If a helper T cell encounters its special molecule in a dangerous situation, it can quickly clone itself to create a mini-army of helper lymphocytes that can attack the molecule more effectively.

• **Regulatory T cells** are peacekeeping lymphocytes. Like the helpers, regulatory lymphocytes are created with expertise about a particular molecule. But their speciality is harmless molecules – those found on our own tissues, on probiotic bacteria in our microflora or on pollen. Regulatory T cells calm things down and protect innocent 'bystanders'. Scientists have only recently discovered that this job is just as important to our health as fighting the bad guys – and that probiotics are involved in T-cell development.

• **B cells**, also known as antibody-producing lymphocytes, are the media experts. They create antibodies, molecules that are the equivalent of 'Wanted' posters to help the other white blood cells to distinguish good guys from bad guys. Like the T cells, B cells specialise. Some produce posters of harmless molecules, which are written in a particular 'language', called sIgA, which is used only for the good guys. These lymphocytes stay in the lining of our internal tube, especially the gut. Other B cells specialise in dangerous molecules; their posters are written in other languages. Once the antibodies are released, they circulate throughout the body. When they encounter their target, they stick to it. Other white blood cells spot the antibody and know whether to treat the target as an enemy.

Phagocytes (Foot Soldiers)

Phagocytes roam the body looking for bad guys to attack. Who's a suspect? Any molecule on a 'Wanted' poster that they can read – and they understand only the languages describing dangerous molecules. They also attack microbes that happen to be near a damaged part of the body, just in case they're responsible for the damage.

When phagocytes spot a suspect, they surround it, eat it, and digest it. And then they die. The word 'phagocyte' comes from the Greek words *phagein,* meaning 'to eat', and *kytos,* meaning 'cell'. Phagocytes are cells that eat. But that's not all they can do. Phagocytes are armed with chemical weapons. They can kill microbes by dumping poisonous chemicals on them.

Sometimes other white blood cells direct the phagocytes. A helper lymphocyte can order phagocytes to attack. Or a regulatory lymphocyte might come upon the scene and send a chemical signal that translates to 'Cool it'.

➤ THE CHEMICAL ARSENAL OF ◀ WHITE BLOOD CELLS

Phagocytes make some of the same chemicals we use to kill germs in our bathrooms. Two examples: hydrogen peroxide and hypochlorous acid (chlorine bleach).

These chemicals are highly toxic. When you use household bleach to disinfect a kitchen counter, the instructions on the bottle tell you to make a greatly diluted solution. But the chemicals that phagocytes release are full-strength. So it's not surprising that nearby tissue may be damaged by them.

Dendritic Cells (Intelligence Agents)

Dendritic cells lurk in every tissue in our body. Their job is to grab molecules and drag them to the T cells, along with a report on whether the molecule was found in an area of damage. The word dendritic is derived from the Greek word for tree, *dendron*. Dendritic cells have tree-like branches, which they use as arms to snatch their prey.

The dendritic cells keep track of what's coming through our digestive tract. They also help train the T cells to either become helper or regulatory lymphocytes. Each T cell is created to have expertise in a particular molecule, but they don't know at first if their molecule is dangerous or harmless. They learn that from the dendritic cells.

If a T cell's molecule turns out to be associated with damage, the T cell becomes a helper lymphocyte. Otherwise, it's a peacekeeping regulatory lymphocyte. The dendritic cells operate mostly in the gut. This is the key to the connection between probiotics and development of inflammation-reducing regulatory lymphocytes.

Mast Cells (Water Brigade)

Mast cells are white blood cells that are equipped with the equivalent of a spanner that opens a fire hose. They mostly live in the parts of our body that are exposed to the outside world – our skin, our respiratory tract and the tube that runs through our digestive tract.

Phagocytes eat and poison intruders, but mast cells prefer to turn the water on them. This makes a lot of sense when the enemy is relatively large. For example, parasites are often too big for phagocytes to destroy. But mast cells can open the fire hose to flush them away. They produce chemicals, such as histamine, that signal fluids to flow in from the blood and flood the mucosa or tissues under the skin. That's helpful when the body is battling an infection and needs to bring in white blood cells. Unfortunately, mast cells sometimes turn on the water to attack harmless particles – thereby creating allergic reactions, such as a runny nose, bronchial congestion or hives.

A Database of Molecules

Throughout our lives, our immune system labours over an extraordinary task: to maintain a vast database of good and bad molecules. That's how our white blood cells know what to attack and what they can safely ignore. Most of this knowledge must be acquired, though we're born with a head start. An infant's immune system can already tell if a molecule is part of its body's own cells and therefore a good guy. It can also recognise damage to tissues; any molecule associated with damage is assumed to be a bad guy.

⨝ HOW VACCINES WORK ⨝

Years ago, parents were grateful if their children developed mild cases of measles, mumps or chickenpox – that meant they were immune from more severe versions of the disease. Now we have vaccines that accomplish the same thing, but without the illness.

A vaccine fools a helper lymphocyte into responding to a harmless microbe that's similar to one that causes a particular disease. Sometimes the vaccine consists of microbes that have been killed chemically or by heat; sometimes weakened forms of the microbe are used.

Either way, the helper lymphocyte produces clones that can attack the microbe. In addition, antibody-producing lymphocytes post its 'mug shot' as a dangerous suspect. If the disease-causing version of the microbe ever appears in the body, the immune system is ready to respond.

A breastfeeding infant gets antibodies from the mother's milk, which helps out until his or her own antibodies develop. Over the years – as we encounter microbes from the environment and from illnesses – our immune system becomes increasingly effective. (That's why small children typically get ill much more frequently than adults do.) The database expands; more and more 'mug shots' are posted. In addition, the specialised helper lymphocytes have cloned themselves every time they address a threat. So our body now contains numerous police teams that have been trained to deal effectively with the microbes that have threatened us in the past.

A SIMPLE IMMUNE RESPONSE

Let's start with a kiss. Congratulations: you've now been exposed to anywhere from just a few microbes to millions of them. (The specific number depends on many factors, such as how passionate the kiss was, and whether antimicrobial mouthwash was involved.) Your mind may be elsewhere at that moment, but your immune system has leapt into action.

Phagocytes, which constantly patrol the body looking for trouble, are on the scene. They recognise some cold viruses and other germs from 'Wanted' posters left by antibody-producing lymphocytes. The phagocytes immediately begin gobbling microbes, using their poisonous chemicals as condiments. After these greedy white blood cells digest their fill, they die. Sorry to mention this, but every time you swallow, you're probably disposing of many dead phagocytes and their microbial meals.

Pretty soon, all the potentially dangerous microbes have been dispatched. There's nothing more to excite the remaining phagocytes. They calm down, go back on patrol and look for the next threat. Incidents like this occur all the time, without you ever noticing them. Meanwhile, thanks to your immune system, you aren't going to catch a cold.

FIGHTING INFECTION WITH INFLAMMATION

Yesterday you were wiping down a picnic table outside and cut your finger on a rusty nail. You washed your hands, put on a plaster, and forgot about it. But now it's very much on your mind. Your finger is swollen, hot and painful – and you're developing a fever. What's happening?

The rusty nail delivered a significant bacterial load when it penetrated your skin. It not only brought microbes from the nail, but also dragged in some *Staphylococcus aureus* that were living on your skin. This bacterium, called Staph for short, is notorious for causing skin infections, such as boils, sties and impetigo.

Our skin produces antimicrobial compounds to protect us against harmful microbes, but these compounds aren't very effective against Staph. All of us carry small amounts of Staph on our skin. Usually it can't get into our body because the skin itself serves as a barrier. But all bets are off if the skin is broken. When that happens, Staph seizes the opportunity to slip inside.

When you cut your finger on the rusty nail, patrolling phagocytes were already there. More were summoned by the broken skin itself – damaged tissue produces hormone-like chemicals that can issue a 999 call. The phagocytes spotted damage to the skin and began trying to eat all the microbes in the wound.

But Staph is tough. Many do not merely survive the initial immune assault, but actually begin to divide and increase in number. The phagocytes realise they're losing this battle, so they summon back-up – literally a call for blood. As the flow of blood to the site increases, the tissues become swollen and hot. This process is called inflammation. By delivering white blood cells to the battlefield, inflammation plays an essential role in the immune response. Casualties – dead microbes and dead white blood cells – pile up, creating the thick yellowish fluid called pus.

At last the Staph is brought under control by the phagocytes. It's about to be eliminated. But wait! Another type of microbe was on that rusty nail, one that the phagocytes haven't been able to kill: *Clostridium tetani*, the bacterium that causes tetanus. *C. tetani* are increasing in numbers and producing a toxin that's really beginning to cause damage. It's time for a new strategy, one that will mount a stronger but more focused attack on this surviving invader. That requires intelligent leadership and more potent weapons. So far I've talked about skirmishes. This is war.

The new leaders, helper T cells, were trained by the dendritic cells and they're much smarter than the phagocytes. They clone themselves, providing more leadership and expertise. Moreover, you've had your tetanus shots. Thus your immune system has been fooled into thinking it has fought this battle with *Clostridium tetani* before. The inflammatory response will be quick and effective.

Meanwhile, the chemicals produced by the immune system during inflammation are starting to affect parts of the body outside the immediate problem area. The immune reaction has caused a fever. That might make you feel dreadful, but it's actually a helpful response. Most germs grow best at normal body temperature, 37°C. A higher temperature is less favourable and slows them down.

As the immune response develops, the helper lymphocytes – clones as well as originals – take over the traffic signals. Reinforcement troops arrive in great numbers and move into the damaged area. The new situation triggers a change in the phagocytes. They become 'activated': it's just like what happened in the old *Marvel* comics when Dr Bruce Banner, nuclear physicist, became enraged and was transformed into the Incredible Hulk. Activated phagocytes can make even more destructive chemicals, including some not found in your bathroom.

The phagocytes use antibodies (their 'Wanted' posters) to identify this dangerous microbe. They also get further directions from the helper T cells in identifying their target. The pumped-up phagocytes dump their toxins only on the tetanus bacteria and not on nearby tissue. Instead of the previous chemical chaos, the immune response is now as precise as surgery.

The regulatory T cells observe the situation. The bacteria are finally losing ground, but the remaining phagocytes and helper T cells are still revved up. They start eyeing harmless molecules, looking for a fight. The regulatory lymphocytes – recognising that the battle is over – send their essential peacekeeping chemical signals. The phagocytes and helper lymphocytes demobilise. The chemical sirens that summon an inflammatory response are turned off. The influx of blood slows; inflammation begins to resolve; the fever subsides. Not only is the skin healed, but thanks to the regulatory lymphocytes, there's no sign of inflammation or infection.

I've just described an inflammatory response in the skin. The same sequence of events occurs throughout our body whenever we're faced with a damage-causing microbe, such as respiratory infection. The immune system can generate inflammation anywhere in the body – in the lungs, sinuses, gut and even in the arteries leading to the heart. It's the responsibility of regulatory T cells to keep inflammatory responses under control. And one of the jobs of probiotics is to help create these essential white blood cells.

AN IMMUNE RESPONSE

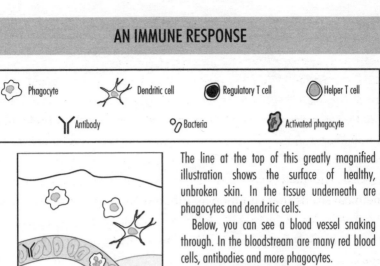

The line at the top of this greatly magnified illustration shows the surface of healthy, unbroken skin. In the tissue underneath are phagocytes and dendritic cells.

Below, you can see a blood vessel snaking through. In the bloodstream are many red blood cells, antibodies and more phagocytes.

Behind the blood vessel is a lymphatic vessel, carrying clear lymph fluid.

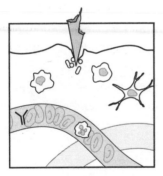

A piece of dirty, rusty metal breaks the skin, bringing along bacteria.

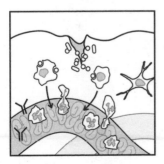

The phagocytes spot damage to the skin and begin eating the bacteria in the wound. More phagocytes are summoned by the damaged tissue.

The flow of blood increases. Phagocytes leave the bloodstream and join the battle. Antibodies join in.

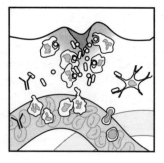

The bacteria divide and increase in number. Many are eaten and destroyed by the phagocytes.

The tissue near the wound becomes inflamed and swollen. As the inflammatory response develops, more phagocytes leave the blood and enter the tissue, accompanied by helper T cells.

Antibodies and dendritic cells help to identify the bacteria to be eliminated.

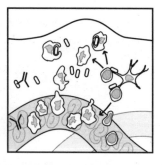

The phagocytes have eliminated one type of bacteria, but another proves more resistant.

With the help of dendritic cells in the tissue, the helper T cells produce chemical signals to activate the phagocytes. They become super microbe destroyers and summon more T cells and phagocytes.

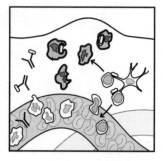

The activated phagocytes eat and destroy all of the remaining bacteria at the site of infection.

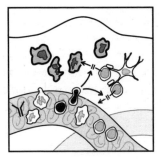

The infection is eliminated.

Regulatory T cells enter the tissue and send peacekeeping signals. These block the activation signals sent by the helper T cells. (Note: if there are not enough regulatory T cells at this step to completely shut down the response, chronic inflammation will develop.)

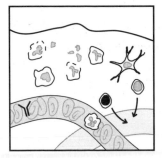

The infection has been destroyed and activation signals for the phagocytes are now blocked by the regulatory T cells.

White blood cells leave the tissue; the flow of blood returns to normal.

Most of the phagocytes have died; the remainder clean up the battlefield. The T cells exit via the lymphatic vessels.

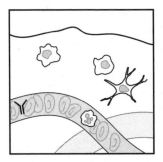

Inflammation has resolved completely. The skin is healed and the tissue shows no sign of infection.

WHAT CAN GO WRONG?

So far I've told two greatly simplified tales, of a kiss and a rusty nail, in which the immune system triumphs over evil. Fortunately, that's what usually happens – which is why most of us are chronically quite healthy rather than chronically ill. But the immune system isn't perfect. And sometimes things go wrong. Here are scenarios that don't have happy endings.

The Database Contains Errors

You're waiting to complete a credit card purchase and suddenly you notice that the shop assistant is giving you nervous looks. Then the manager appears and asks you to step into her office. It turns out that the credit card company's records indicate that your card was stolen in an armed robbery – and to make matters even worse, the description of the thief sounds exactly like you. You're an upstanding citizen with a perfect credit history, but there's been a data entry error and an unfortunate coincidence.

Our immune system's database makes record-keeping errors, too. When that happens, we're in trouble. If the mistake involves classifying a harmful molecule as safe, the result might be illness – including cancer (see the box on the next page). Problems also ensue when a harmless molecule goes into the database as a dangerous one, and the full fury of our immune reactions lands upon the innocent. Possible consequences range from mild allergies to life-threatening autoimmune disorders – and all the conditions, known and not yet known, that are caused by unnecessary inflammation.

Autoimmune Diseases

If the immune system's database mistakenly flags one of our own cells as a threat, our body attacks itself. This is the kind of mistake that causes autoimmune disorders, including rheumatoid arthritis, type 1 diabetes, multiple sclerosis and many other conditions.

For example, in type 1 diabetes, the immune system decides that the insulin-producing beta cells in the pancreas are dangerous and does everything in its considerable power to wipe them out. Why does this terrible mistake occur? The leading hypothesis is that type 1 diabetes follows an immune response to a viral infection, in which the regulatory response is inadequate. Candidate

CANCER: A FAILURE TO RECOGNISE DANGER FROM WITHIN

Cancer is actually many different diseases. But all of them start with cells from our own body whose DNA has been damaged. As a result of this damage, the cells have become abnormal versions of themselves – an abnormal breast cell in the case of breast cancer, an abnormal colon cell if it's colon cancer. These defective cells can't perform the functions of their normal counterparts; they also proliferate out of control.

A vigilant immune system can recognise cancerous cells and destroy them. But as you might guess, it's trickier to recognise danger in cells that closely resemble healthy ones. Because of this, the immune system sometimes gives cancer cells a free pass and allows them to grow. People who have compromised immune systems, such as those with AIDS or those taking immunosuppressive drugs, are at elevated risk for cancer.

viruses include Coxsackie B virus and other enteroviruses, which can cause flu-like illnesses, viral meningitis and other acute diseases. These viruses can look a lot like the pancreas's own beta cells.

Disastrous consequences flow from this unfortunate coincidence plus a poor regulatory response. When the immune system eliminates the virus, the regulatory cells are supposed to call off the troops and make sure they don't go after anything else. But that doesn't happen. The immune system continues its search for the virus, but there are no more viruses to attack. At this point, the helper T cells decide that a molecule on the beta cells looks like a molecule on the virus they were just battling. Now the beta cells become the target. The misguided immune system attack eventually destroys the beta cells, leaving the body with no way to make insulin. Until insulin treatment was developed in the 1920s – one of the great advances of modern medicine – type 1 diabetes meant certain death.

We don't fully understand the underlying causes of auto-immunity. But it's possible that almost all autoimmune diseases start in this way: with a case of mistaken identity, something that immunologists refer to as molecular mimicry. If so, the healthy functioning of regulatory lymphocytes holds the answer to preventing and possibly even treating many autoimmune diseases. For example, we can't prevent or cure type 1 diabetes today; all we can do is compensate for it with insulin injections. But if we could find or create regulatory T cells that identify beta cells as harmless, perhaps we could grow lots of them, put them back in the body – and save the beta cells.

Allergies

Allergic reactions are the result of yet another immune system mistake. They occur when the immune system's database classifies innocuous particles from the environment – allergens – as threats. The particle could be a perfectly healthy food. Or it might be something we inhale, such as pollen, cat dander, mould spores or dust mites. How does such a mistake occur? The underlying problem is that the antibody-producing lymphocytes, the B cells, signal that the allergens should be considered dangerous.

As I mentioned before, the antibody-producing lymphocytes create their 'Wanted' posters in the equivalent of several different languages. Phagocytes understand languages that mast cells don't comprehend, and vice versa. The signals for allergens are in a language that scientists call IgE. (Ig stands for 'immunoglobulin', which is another word for 'antibody'.) IgE is understood by mast cells, but not by phagocytes. Signals for germs, on the other hand, are in languages that phagocytes comprehend, but mast cells don't. Yet another language, called secretory IgA (or sIgA), is used exclusively to identify harmless molecules.

An allergic response – the kind produced by mast cells in response to an IgE antibody – is different in some ways from immune responses involving phagocytes, the cells that eat microbes and dump chemicals on them. Mast cells are the ones that open the fire hoses. In an allergic response, the mast cells are trying to wash away the problem. They do this by releasing a chemical called histamine, which produces the classic allergic symptoms of runny nose and watery eyes. Regulatory cells, ever the peacekeepers, counter these effects by decreasing IgE production. That's why probiotics can help keep allergic responses in check.

Inflammation Persists

Inflammation is a powerful force for healing. However, we're now beginning to understand that chronic inflammation – a response that continues when it's not needed – has devastating effects upon the entire body.

Tissue Damage

In the story of the rusty nail, the phagocytes and helper T cells would have continued their attack – even in the absence of the tetanus bacteria – if it hadn't been for the regulatory T cells. The powerful toxic chemicals released by the phagocytes would have splashed on surrounding cells, causing damage. Remember that damaged tissues make 999 calls, summoning more white blood cells and leading to even more damage. The situation would have spiralled out of control. This is exactly what happens in auto-immune diseases, such as inflammatory bowel disease, where a mistaken immune response destroys part of the intestines.

Effects of Inflammation Outside the Immune System

Few people realise that when they come down with the flu, most of their discomfort – fever, fatigue, muscle pain, a headache – is not caused by the virus itself. Rather, these symptoms are produced by the immune system as it fights that virus. The same is true for just about all disease symptoms.

We've long suspected that at least some of these effects are built into the immune response for a reason. For example, as I mentioned above, a fever can help destroy harmful microbes. Some have speculated that fatigue could be useful because it persuades you to rest. That permits the body to focus its energy on fighting germs rather than on activities like playing tennis. But what's the point of muscular aches and pains? Why should we feel so dreadful while the immune system is at war? I wish I could give you an answer, but we simply don't know.

What we *do* know is that the immune system is central to proper functioning of all parts of the body. Some of the most exciting recent discoveries in immunology involve previously unsuspected connections between the immune responses and other systems, such as the digestive system, respiratory system and nervous system. It turns out that many of the signalling chemicals our body makes for other purposes actually communicate with the immune system, too. This means that in an emergency, the immune system can use chemical signals to issue orders to other systems – it's like declaring martial law and giving the police authority over civilians.

For example, our nerve cells make chemicals, including neurotransmitters, that can influence sleep and eating behaviour, cause pain, and even affect mood. During an inflammatory response, the immune system can take over and alter production of these chemicals. Thus inflammation that's seemingly confined to one part of the body can generate whole-body effects, including fatigue and generalised muscle aches. What's more, inflammation-related changes in neurotransmitters can produce emotional responses: depression, anxiety and irritability. When we have the flu, it's not just the headache and nausea that make us feel so miserable; neurotransmitters are at work, too – thanks to the immune system.

THE CASE OF THE RESTLESS MICE

Early in my career, I worked on a series of experiments with special mice that had been bred to lack a key immune system molecule that signals danger. Because of this genetic defect, these mice were vulnerable to certain diseases. During this period, I attended a seminar given by other immunologists who were working with the same mice. I expected to hear about experiments in which these susceptible mice had been infected with various disease organisms. But what struck me most at that seminar was an aside from one of the scientists. He said, 'By the way, these mice need less sleep than their normal counterparts.'

Why was this so striking? Sleep cycles are controlled by the nervous system, not by the immune system. This was the first time I'd ever heard about immune system signal molecules having an effect on other systems.

This phenomenon of dual effects – a single chemical that can communicate both with the immune system and with some other system of the body – is now an area of great interest among scientists. And I'm not just talking about immunologists. I often hear from other specialists who say, 'Hey! I found your molecule in my system.' The implications are exciting. One widely held hypothesis is that chronic low-level inflammation could account for baffling conditions – such as irritable bowel syndrome, chronic fatigue and fibromyalgia – that are characterised by multiple seemingly unconnected symptoms.

THE UNSUNG HEROES: REGULATORY LYMPHOCYTES

The problems I've just described – autoimmune diseases, allergies, out-of-control inflammation – have a single cause: regulatory T cells didn't do their job. Either they didn't develop properly, or they didn't develop in sufficient numbers to counterbalance the activities of the helper T cells.

Until about ten years ago, we didn't know all that much about regulatory lymphocytes. The problem was that there aren't nearly as many of them as there are of helper lymphocytes. So they were hard to find under a standard microscope. This obstacle disappeared with the development of a new technology called flow cytometry, which allows us to send a parade of cells, one by one, past a very thin beam of light. This light (usually a laser) can make certain cells glow; we can also sort them by types.

Over the past five years, as flow cytometry permitted us to learn more about regulatory lymphocytes, they've become a focus of intense research in immunology. The implications for treatment are especially exciting. For instance, rheumatoid arthritis is an autoimmune disease caused by errant white blood cells that attack the cells lining the joints. If we could work out a way to stimulate development of regulatory T cells that identify joint cells as harmless, we might be able to stop the inflammatory process from within. We then could cure the disease instead of merely treating it with painkillers and immunosuppressant drugs, such as corticosteroids.

HOW PROBIOTICS PROMOTE A HEALTHY IMMUNE SYSTEM

The complex relationship between probiotics and the immune system is a topic of enormous interest and research activity at major medical centres around the world. My department at the

University of Michigan is creating a new research centre that focuses exclusively on the interaction between our microflora and our immune and digestive systems. Several new faculty members have been recruited for this work.

This much we already know: our body needs a balance between regulatory and helper lymphocytes for the immune system to function optimally. As we unravel the incredibly complicated process by which this balance is achieved, the crucial role of probiotics becomes clearer.

T cells are born in the bone marrow and receive a preliminary education in the thymus. After they leave the thymus, some are destined to become helper T cells; others will be regulatory T cells. This final transformation can occur anywhere in the body. But it happens most often in the gut, following an encounter with a dendritic cell – a cell that trains lymphocytes to be helper or regulatory cells. If a dendritic cell finds a molecule in an area with damage signals, it assumes that this molecule is harmful and creates a helper T cell.

Things turn out differently when probiotics get involved. First, probiotics promote a healthy gut – one that isn't damaged. They do this by producing antimicrobial compounds that destroy harmful microbes. And they also crowd out the undesirables by competing with them for nutrients. Second, probiotics can actually send 'all is well' chemical messages to the dendritic cells. Together, these effects of probiotics mean that the dendritic cells in the gut are more likely to get a favourable impression of the molecules they grab. As a result, more lymphocytes turn into regulatory T cells, nature's own way of fighting inflammation.

Probiotics also affect B cells in the intestinal tract. In the presence of probiotics, the B cells are more likely to make secretory IgA (the antibodies that declare molecules to be harmless) than IgE (antibodies that activate mast cells). The result is fewer allergic responses to innocuous substances.

My laboratory at the University of Michigan is looking into another intriguing possibility: that there may be 'regulatory phagocytes' – phagocytes that don't simply eat harmful microbes but that develop at sites of inflammation and act like regulatory T cells. If so, our next question will be whether probiotics help to stimulate development of these special phagocytes.

We now understand that probiotics do much more than promote the health of our gut. They also foster profoundly important changes in our white blood cells. That means an immune system that serves us, rather than harms us.

The first four chapters of this book have provided a crash course in microbiology and immunology. Now that you understand the basics, it's time to move out of the laboratory and into real life. What does all this mean for your health? How do probiotics actually help to prevent and treat disease? In Part 2, you'll tour the front lines of the probiotic revolution, where research is coming up with some extraordinary answers.

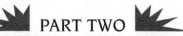

PART TWO

Preventing and Treating Disease

We cannot solve our problems with the same thinking we used when we created them.

— ALBERT EINSTEIN

Introduction

A few years ago, when I first considered using probiotics to relieve my lifelong allergies and asthma, I scoured all available research reports. What I read left me both excited and frustrated. On one hand, many studies were extremely promising. But on the other, research was incomplete. In some cases, findings were limited to animals – or even bacteria in test tubes. Different investigations sometimes produced conflicting evidence. Instead of the large-scale, well-controlled clinical trials that are the 'gold standard' for proving that treatments are effective, I usually found small pilot studies.

Though medical research on probiotics has exploded since then, it's still at an early stage. As you read this section of the book, which reviews what we know now about the therapeutic value of probiotics, you may experience the same combination of excitement and frustration that I did.

You probably have many practical questions about using probiotics to improve your health – especially if you suffer from a chronic condition like inflammatory bowel disease, allergies or an autoimmune disorder. You may be wondering which probiotics are most effective against a particular disease. What dose should be used? How long do they take to produce improvements?

Medical investigators are asking these questions, too. But scientific progress can seem frustratingly slow when you want answers *now*. So I want to explain why the time-consuming preliminaries – the animal studies and even the contradictory findings – are necessary parts of the process. And I also want to reassure you that you don't have to wait before reaping the benefits of these remarkable friendly microbes.

IN SEARCH OF SCIENTIFIC PROOF

It's surprisingly difficult to prove that a medical treatment really works in people. Human beings are very complicated, and a wide variety of factors could account for any observed improvement. In designing a study, scientists must try to control as many of these factors as possible. But they can't account for all of them. For instance, scientists usually can't control the stress levels in subjects' lives, the food they eat or how much they sleep – all of which affect health.

Ethical issues also limit scientific research in humans. We can't inflict chronic diseases upon healthy subjects. Even if we're testing a cure, we can't compel people to join (or to remain in) clinical studies – or to follow investigators' instructions. That's why medical journal reports often must acknowledge that dropouts and imperfect participant compliance may cast doubt upon their findings.

Small wonder that researchers first turn to laboratory animals to study disease and treatments. We can start with genetically identical animals and give all of them the same disease at the same time. Any factors in their environment that might be relevant to treatment can be strictly controlled: it's simple to house them in identical cages, expose them to the same amount of light and darkness and keep them on the same diet. If a probiotic strain can successfully treat laboratory animals with a particular disease, that doesn't necessarily mean that this probiotic will work in people. However, it's a hopeful sign that justifies the effort required to perform a human study.

One thing that's common to human and animal studies of probiotics is that they usually test just one strain of bacteria at a time. This allows researchers to determine what's actually effective. But it also reduces the odds of successful treatment – and it helps to explain why some studies of probiotics have had disappointing or conflicting results. The answer could be as simple as trying a different bacterial strain or dose. Or it could be more complex, such as needing to combine more than one type of probiotic to see an effect.

WHY YOU CAN USE PROBIOTICS NOW

In the following chapters, I'll describe the latest research on using probiotics to prevent and treat chronic diseases. Sometimes they're successful on their own; sometimes they work together with existing medical therapies, boosting their effectiveness or reducing their side effects.

Even by the very conservative standards of mainstream science, evidence for probiotics is already strong in many cases. Despite the fact that other evidence is preliminary or confusing, one message is clear: we know that probiotics are safe. The fermented foods that are rich in probiotics, such as yoghurt, have been part of the human diet for thousands of years. Moreover, the 'doses' that have been found effective in medical studies – typically, the equivalent of a serving or two of yoghurt per day – are completely consistent with what's recommended for healthy eating by well-established nutritional guidelines. This is not like taking potentially toxic megadoses of vitamin pills.

We also know a great deal about how probiotics work in the body. Their promise comes from basic scientific research as well as from treatment studies. As I explained in Chapter 4, there's a clear relationship between a balanced microflora in the digestive tract and proper functioning of the immune system. We know that probiotic bacteria can correct misguided inflammatory responses, and we also know that such inflammatory responses underlie many chronic diseases. With such links firmly established, there's excellent reason to have confidence in the therapeutic benefits of these friendly bacteria.

When I decided to introduce probiotics into my diet, I couldn't be sure my allergies and asthma would improve as a result. But I felt the experiment was well worth trying. Moreover, I knew that it involved no risk. Nor was I ignoring medical advice: I was prepared to continue using the medications my doctor had prescribed for my allergies and asthma – antihistamines and an inhaler as needed. As it turned out, I seldom need them any more. A month after I began using probiotics, my previously severe mould allergies had been tamed. Since my asthma was allergy-related, attacks became rare. To this day, I include probiotics in my diet, as do my wife and two children.

If you suffer from one or more of the chronic conditions discussed in this section, the research I report may offer you important new options. Talk to your GP about incorporating probiotics into your treatment plan. If scientists have already confirmed that a specific probiotic is effective, that's a logical place to start. Otherwise, a good strategy is to consume a variety of probiotics.

The best medicine, of course, is preventive medicine. Probiotics aren't just for people who are ill or at risk. There's considerable evidence that they can help to optimise well-being for those fortunate enough to enjoy good health. The probiotic revolution includes all of us!

CHAPTER FIVE

Optimising Health with Probiotics

You're on a crowded plane, and half the passengers are sneezing and coughing. Or maybe the 24-hour flu is going round at work. Or perhaps you ate that egg salad too quickly, not realising that one of the ingredients was *salmonella*. Malicious microbes are on the prowl. Will you be among their victims – or one of the lucky ones who manage to escape? The answer depends in part upon the microbial balance in your GI (gastrointestinal) tract.

All of us are exposed to germs; all of us are battered by stress, at least occasionally. Research shows that probiotics keep our immune system combat-ready. At every stage of life – from before birth to old age – probiotics help us to remain healthy.

PROMOTING WELLNESS

Healthcare sometimes seems like a game of catch-up. We go to our GP when something goes wrong, hoping for a solution. Even if we're diligent about getting check-ups, their focus is usually on screening for disease. But of course, what we really want is to keep healthy. That requires a strong, balanced, and resilient immune system – one that can ward off the many everyday threats to our health and help us to bounce back quickly from the inevitable occasional illness.

PROBIOTICS IN EVERYDAY PRACTICE

Jay Sandweiss, DO, is an osteopathic physician who is board-certified in neuromusculoskeletal medicine, osteopathic manipulative medicine and medical acupuncture. He teaches continuing medical education courses nationally and internationally, and has a thriving medical practice in Ann Arbor, Michigan. On the subject of probiotics for everyday health, he comments:

I have an integrated medical practice in which I combine Western medicine with evidence-based complementary and alternative therapies. I often recommend probiotics to my patients to keep their health 'bank account' full in the event that they need to draw from it when problems occur. Probiotics serve a preventive and protective role, and they act as a repair force in keeping my patients healthy. I also use probiotics to treat patients suffering from dysbiosis, an imbalance of gastrointestinal functions or microbial populations that can result from body stresses including – to name a few – GI infections, dietary 'indiscretions', various nutrient deficiencies and taking certain medications, including antibiotics and non-steroidal anti-inflammatory drugs, such as aspirin and ibuprofen.

Including probiotics in your diet is like taking your car in for its annual MOT before things go wrong. You may recall from Chapter 2 that probiotic microbes wipe out germs directly by successfully competing with them for nutrients and a prime location in the gut. Chapter 4 explained how probiotics can boost immune-system functioning by minimising inflammation. That's important because many symptoms of illness are produced by inflammation, and not by the disease-causing microbes themselves.

Now, research outside the laboratory, involving people in everyday settings, is demonstrating that people who take probiotics enjoy a wellness advantage. In Chapter 1, I described a report from Sweden finding that workers who were given probiotics had fewer illness-related absences than colleagues who received a placebo. Think of the workers in the placebo group: all of them considered themselves healthy – that was a requirement to join the study. Yet the experiment demonstrated that they could have been even healthier with probiotics.

A recent investigation in Germany recruited 479 healthy adults aged 18 to 67. All were given nutritional supplements with vitamins and minerals. But half were chosen at random to receive lookalike supplements that also contained several probiotics in the *Lactobacillus* and *Bifidobacterium* genera. Neither the investigators nor the participants themselves knew which supplements they were getting. Over the three-month study period – which took place during the winter and spring cold season – participants were asked to keep a daily health diary. Any cold symptoms or fevers were recorded. Those who caught colds filled out questionnaires detailing the severity of their runny noses, scratchy throats, coughs, headaches, muscle pains, conjunctivitis, fatigue and loss of appetite. A subgroup of 122 volunteers also received medical tests to determine how well their immune systems were functioning and to make sure the probiotics had colonised their digestive tract (indeed, they had).

The results should encourage anyone who would like to minimise the annoyance of the common cold. Those whose supplements contained probiotics weren't cold-free. But their colds were shorter by an average of almost two days, and their symptoms were significantly less severe. Should credit go to improved immune-system functioning? Yes. In the subgroup that received additional tests, white blood cell counts were higher among those taking supplements with probiotics. These findings were published in a leading medical journal, *Clinical Nutrition*, in 2005.

BUFFERING THE EFFECTS OF STRESS

Stress is part of life. Up to a point, it's actually good for us. If we're strolling through the zoo and happen to encounter an escaped boa constrictor, there's nothing like a stress power surge to get us moving in the opposite direction. Stress can help us to deal with danger; it can rev us up when we need to perform. Under the right circumstances, we might even enjoy the hyper-alert, heart-pounding sensations caused by emotional stress. Just ask the people standing in a queue at a funfair roller coaster. Or a person newly in love. Stress that produces positive effects is sometimes called 'eustress', in contrast to the bad kind, 'distress'.

When our nervous system picks up signs of physical or emotional distress, it signals for the release of stress hormones and chemical messengers, called neurotransmitters, which speed to other parts of the body. That's why our heart rate increases when we're frightened and our stomach tightens when we're anxious or upset. Even low-level stress, if chronic, can produce physical symptoms because of the constant infusion of stress hormones. Examples include tension headaches, high blood pressure and digestive difficulties. In addition, some research has linked chronic stress to life-threatening conditions like cardiovascular disease and cancer.

Now we're learning that there may be yet another reason to get stressed about chronic stress: the negative impact of stress-related neurotransmitters on the gut microflora. For example, some strains of the potentially harmful bacteria *E. coli* grow faster in a culture flask if the flask contains the stress hormones epinephrine (adrenaline) or norepinephrine (noradrenaline). It turns out that human norepinephrine is very similar to a chemical that bacteria use to signal their presence to other nearby bacteria. When *E. coli* receive these signals, they undergo biochemical changes that make them more harmful to us.

Some scientists now speculate that when we're stressed and all these hormones are released, our nervous system inadvertently starts 'talking' to our gut microbes. These signals may tell some bacteria to multiply and direct others to limit their growth. The intestinal tract contains the largest number of nerves of any part of the body except the brain. The more stress we experience, the more stress hormones our body releases – and the greater the possible effect on our gut microbes.

Stress has the potential to tip our microfloral balance away from probiotics – which also affects the balance of regulatory versus helper T cells. As a result, the immune system will regulate itself less effectively, leading to increased inflammation in the body. Scientists already know that some stress hormones can affect the immune system directly. So perhaps the combination of direct and indirect (via the gut microflora) effects on the immune system explains why chronic inflammatory diseases are more prevalent in 'stressed-out' cultures like ours than elsewhere in the world.

Research suggests that probiotics can help to counter stress. No, probiotic foods and supplements won't save us from rush-hour traffic and unreasonable relatives. But evidence is growing that probiotics can protect us from at least some of the damaging physical effects of stress – including effects on our gut and our immune system.

One of the first studies to link human stress, the immune system and probiotics was performed by Spanish scientists. How did they ensure that participants were under stress? They recruited university students who were about to undergo three weeks of exams. They knew from prior research that academic stress suppresses immune response. Now they wanted to determine if a cultured milk drink containing probiotics could help.

Over a six-week period that began three weeks before exams, 73 volunteers received the probiotic beverage; a control group of 63 students drank ordinary milk. Their anxiety levels and their white blood cells were measured at the start of the study and again at the end. As expected, anxiety went up as exams approached. White blood cell counts, representing immune function, showed the predictable decline in the students who drank plain milk. But those who consumed probiotics actually improved their immune status – despite the fact that they were just as emotionally stressed as the control group. The findings were published in the *European Journal of Nutrition* in 2004.

PROBIOTICS THROUGH THE LIFE CYCLE

We benefit from probiotics throughout our lives. However, our needs change over time, as we move from one stage to another. And just as we encounter certain predictable problems, probiotics may provide solutions.

Mums-to-be

When you're pregnant, you're not just eating for two. If you count your gut microbes, you're eating for trillions! And what's good for your microflora is good for you and your baby as well.

CONSUMING PROBIOTICS DURING PREGNANCY

Research hasn't yet established how to optimise the benefits of probiotics during pregnancy – which particular microbes are best and exactly how much of them to consume. But you can't go wrong by following the nutrition guidelines your GP provides.

Dietary recommendations for mums-to-be typically call for four servings of dairy foods per day. If you select fermented products like yoghurt and aged cheese for some of your dairy portions, you'll get plenty of probiotics. Also on the usual lists of recommended foods are fruit, vegetables and whole grains. Many of these contain prebiotics, notably fibre and other components that support probiotic microbes.

What about probiotic supplements? As with all medications taken when you're pregnant – including other supplements as well as prescription and over-the-counter medication – get an okay from your healthcare provider before you take them.

Dealing with Digestive Problems

Gastrointestinal complaints are common during pregnancy. Some difficulties result from the increase in progesterone levels. While this hormone is essential for maintaining a healthy pregnancy, it relaxes the muscles that normally move food through the digestive tract. One consequence is constipation. Other problems are caused by crowding as the growing baby occupies more space in the abdomen. For example, intestinal gas may be more uncomfortable, because the intestines have no room to expand as they would normally do to accommodate it.

Based on our current knowledge, it seems likely that probiotics – especially *Bifidobacteria* – could help. We know, for example, that *Bifidobacteria* can stimulate peristalsis, the contractions of the intestinal muscles that keep things moving. Fruit, vegetables and whole grains – all high in fibre, a prebiotic that supports probiotics – are often recommended to pregnant women to counter constipation. One suggestion if you and your healthcare provider decide you should add probiotics or fibre: introduce them slowly. Both can sometimes cause a temporary increase in gas at first. In Chapter 14, I'll explain simple ways to deal with this.

Preventing Vaginal and Urinary Tract Infections

Pregnant women are more vulnerable to these infections because of hormone-related changes in the microflora. For example, yeast gets a boost from oestrogen, so it proliferates during pregnancy. Normally, *Lactobacillus* keeps yeast in check. But thanks to extra oestrogen, the yeast are better able to compete.

Yeast infections don't harm the baby, though they can be uncomfortable for the mother. Bacterial vaginal infections, on the other hand, aren't merely unpleasant; they also increase the risk of premature birth. As I'll explain in Chapter 8, there's evidence that certain probiotics help to prevent both types of infections by countering the harmful yeasts and bacteria that can cause them. That's great news for any woman who's been plagued by these problems in the past and who's hoping to avoid them during pregnancy. If she does develop a bacterial infection and must take antibiotics, probiotics are a valuable adjunct to treatment: they can head off possible side effects – including *Candida* infections and antibiotic-associated diarrhoea – by boosting the body's army of friendly microbes.

An Infant's New Microflora

The womb is a sterile environment. In fact, should microbes invade it, the mother's immune response might cause premature labour. A newborn emerges into the world without a microflora. But at that moment, microbes enter its body and the infant begins a lifetime of learning to live with them.

Babies born vaginally receive their first exposure to microbes during delivery. The vaginal tract contains a microflora, including the probiotic *Lactobacillus*, which enters the baby's mouth and is swallowed. (This provides yet another reason for an expectant mother to consume probiotics during pregnancy: she can optimise the microflora that greets her baby as it's born.) An infant born via Caesarean section doesn't receive microbes from its mother's vagina. However, all newborns are exposed to microbes at birth: from the instruments and equipment used, from contact with the mother and others present at delivery and from the first breath of air.

What's most important for an infant's developing microflora is the feeding method. The mother's mammary gland ducts become colonised by probiotic microbes, which she can pass along to her baby during breastfeeding. Breast milk contains several compounds that inhibit disease-causing bacteria and promote probiotics. A breastfed baby's gut microflora consists mainly of *Bacteroides* and the probiotic *Bifidobacteria*. In contrast, the gut microflora of a formula-fed baby has fewer of these microbes and a greater array of other microbes, both beneficial and potentially harmful. While the implications of this difference are not yet fully clear, most scientific evidence suggests that infants whose microflora consists mainly of probiotics have lower rates of allergies and asthma. In Chapter 7, I'll describe Finnish research showing that early consumption of probiotics can help to prevent allergies in children.

Both of my children had frequent colds and occasional episodes of diarrhoea or fever when they were babies. If they were exposed to it, they caught it. As an immunologist, I shouldn't have been surprised that they got ill often. Babies' developing immune systems are still learning to cope with germs. Remembering those years, I've been particularly impressed by the strong research findings on the benefits of probiotics for infants.

PROBIOTICS FOR INFANTS?

The best way for an infant to get probiotics is from its mother's milk. The World Health Organization recommends that infants be breastfed exclusively for the first six months of life, if possible. However, formula is sometimes needed for all or part of a baby's diet. Manufacturers are beginning to produce baby formulas supplemented with probiotics and prebiotics. (See Chapter 12, page 281 for information on formulas with prebiotics.)

Early evidence suggests that adding probiotics offers important health advantages to babies who are bottle-fed. However, further research is needed to confirm the benefits and to learn which particular probiotics are most helpful. In the meantime, talk to your baby's paediatrician before making any changes in formula. It's helpful to bring in a label or a bottle of the product that interests you so that the doctor can read the list of ingredients.

Many paediatricians consider yoghurt an excellent option for babies who are eating solid foods – but ask your child's own doctor what's best. Similarly, consult the doctor before giving probiotic supplements to your baby.

Avoiding Illness

As every parent knows, babies exposed to other babies – whether in informal play groups or in more formal settings like childcare facilities – are especially vulnerable to illness. Israeli researchers studied 261 formula-fed infants, aged 4 months to 10 months old, who attended childcare centres. The babies in this study were assigned at random to receive either a regular formula without probiotics or the same formula supplemented with either *Bifidobacterium lactis* (BB-12) or *Lactobacillus reuteri* (American Type

Culture Collection 55730). Over the next twelve weeks, the babies' health was carefully monitored. The results were reported in 2005 in *Pediatrics*: infants who received one of the probiotic-supplemented formulas had fewer bouts of fever and diarrhoea than those who received plain formula. Babies given *L. reuteri* experienced the same benefits plus additional ones: fewer visits to the GP, fewer childcare absences and fewer antibiotic prescriptions.

The second study I want to tell you about was performed by researchers from Johns Hopkins University in Maryland, USA. They recruited 131 healthy infants and toddlers who were attending daycare centres in the Baltimore area. Participants were assigned at random to one of three groups. Two groups received formula supplemented with *Bifidobacterium lactis* and *Streptococcus thermophilus*; one group's formula contained a higher dose of these probiotics than the other. The third group, the controls, received plain formula without probiotic bacteria. Over a period of months – until the babies left daycare or stopped drinking formula – the investigators contacted parents weekly to ask about their child's health. In addition, daycare attendance records were checked and the babies were weighed and measured monthly.

Most investigations of probiotics last only a few months; the twelve-week Israeli study is typical. But the Johns Hopkins researchers particularly wanted to learn whether probiotics would be tolerated over longer periods. Children in their study were followed for an average of seven months. The results were encouraging: formulas containing probiotics were well accepted, even at relatively high doses. The youngsters who consumed probiotics required less healthcare attention and received antibiotics significantly less frequently. These findings were published in the *American Journal of Clinical Nutrition* in 2004. But what really caught my attention in the Johns Hopkins study was this: babies who consumed probiotic formula were significantly less likely to have colic.

Preventing Colic

My wife and I brought our daughter, our first child, home from hospital when she was three days old. We were thrilled. At 9.00 p.m. that first night, we put her down in her cot and she fell asleep immediately. Obviously, she was a wonder child and we were wonder parents. We went to sleep that night very pleased with ourselves. A few hours later, the wonder child introduced us to colic.

Our daughter had colic for four months. By day, she was a happy, delightful infant. Then every night, starting at about 10.00 p.m., the screaming began. The paediatrician assured us that the problem would go away eventually. In the meantime, she gave us a list of tricks to try, with no promises that any of them would work.

We developed a routine. My wife took the first shift, which went until about 2.00 a.m., while I attempted to get some sleep. Then it was my turn. I remember one night when our daughter was about two weeks old. She'd gone to sleep briefly thanks to my wife's efforts, but woke up at 2.15 a.m., screaming. After two weeks of increasing sleep deprivation, I could barely drag myself out of bed. But I picked her up, wrapped her securely in a blanket – swaddling was one of the paediatrician's suggestions – sat down in a rocking chair and attempted to rock her to sleep. No joy. I got up and walked around the room with her. After about half an hour of alternately walking and rocking, her crying finally subsided. With a sense of accomplishment, I brought her to the cot. The moment I put her on the mattress, the screaming resumed.

I tried everything I could think of to console her – simethicone drops, nappy changes, feeding, burping, cuddling, bouncing, rocking, walking, singing, you name it. Nothing worked. Her little face was red from screaming. I carried her into the living room and sat down, completely exhausted. The room was dark, except for the blue light on the video telling me that it was 4.00 a.m. For a moment, I wondered why I'd ever thought that parenthood would enrich my life.

If you've dealt with a colicky infant, you know how miserable it is – and not just for the baby. So I've been fascinated to read about research suggesting that probiotics could help. A team in Turin, Italy, has conducted a series of investigations on colic and the microflora. One of their first discoveries was that colicky infants have different patterns of gut microflora than their non-colicky peers. Those with colic are less frequently colonised by *Lactobacillus* bacteria and more likely to host non-probiotic bacteria. A long-term study by the same group found that colicky infants were more vulnerable to allergies, including allergic rhinitis, conjunctivitis, asthmatic bronchitis, hay fever, atopic eczema and food allergies. As I'll explain in more detail in Chapter 7, all of these conditions have microflora connections.

The Italian group has shown that probiotics and prebiotics can significantly relieve infant colic. In a study published in the *European Journal of Clinical Nutrition* in 2006, involving 199 babies with colic, a prebiotics-laced formula outperformed the combination of a regular formula and simethicone drops, the standard colic treatment. More recently, the Italians described an exciting preliminary study, not yet published, designed to see if probiotics could help. They recruited 68 infants whose bouts of crying lasted for three or more hours daily, three or more days per week, over a period of more than three weeks. (My daughter would have qualified easily.) Half of the babies received drops containing the probiotic *Lactobacillus reuteri*; the rest received simethicone. After four weeks, the conventionally treated infants were still crying for an average of 2 hours and 27 minutes per day. But in striking contrast, those who received the *L. reuteri* drops were down to an average of just 17 minutes of crying per day, which is well within the range of normal. If I could travel back in time to my daughter's infancy, I'd definitely try them!

Keeping Kids Healthy

The microflora evolves as a baby develops from a child into an adult. The first major change occurs with the switch from breast milk or formula to solid foods. This brings a wider variety of microbes into the body and makes the gut microflora more diverse. However, if the youngster's diet is poor – for instance, low in fruit and vegetables and high in sugar – the population of probiotic microbes may decline.

Healthy children, like babies and adults, can become even healthier with probiotics. Especially encouraging are studies of youngsters in group childcare settings. It turns out that probiotics can help to control the minor illnesses that often bounce from one child to another. For example, Finnish researchers recruited 571 healthy children aged 1 to 6 years old who were attending daycare centres in Helsinki. During a seven-month period, half of them were assigned at random to receive milk that contained the probiotic *Lactobacillus rhamnosus* GG, while the rest received plain milk. Until the end of the study, neither the investigators nor the children nor their parents knew which beverage each child was drinking. Meanwhile, researchers kept track of any respiratory or gastrointestinal symptoms, illness-related absences and antibiotics prescriptions. The results, published in the *British Medical Journal* in 2001: children in the *Lactobacillus* group had significantly fewer absences, fewer and less severe respiratory tract infections and fewer antibiotic treatments.

Adulthood

Our body's systems generally work best in young adulthood. I'm sure I'm not the only one who looks back and marvels at how effortless it was to stay vigorous and healthy when I was in my teens, twenties and even thirties. People that age can neglect the basics – diet, exercise, sleep – and seemingly get away with it. But they may be running up health debts that will come back to haunt them sooner or later. By middle age, most of us realise that we can't take good health for granted: we have to work at it.

Over the years, our bodies change in many ways – including the composition of our gut microflora. The major differences, which begin in midlife, involve a decrease in members of the probiotic *Bifidobacterium* genus and an increase in *E. coli* and *Clostridia*. *E. coli* can perform useful functions in the gut – they help to compete against harmful microbes; they make certain vitamins that we absorb. On the other hand, if they leave the GI tract, they can cause disease. Many species of *Clostridia* are just plain bad news. If their numbers get out of control, they can cause serious illnesses. Members of the *Clostridium* genus are responsible for tetanus, botulism and gangrene, as well as antibiotic-associated diarrhoea.

Though we don't have detailed evidence about the consequences of these microbial changes, it seems reasonable to assume that they're not favourable for health. Fortunately, age doesn't diminish the benefits of probiotics.

Improving Digestive Function

A senior citizen once quipped, 'Everything that works hurts. And what doesn't hurt doesn't work.' For many older people, the digestive tract would rank high on both lists – what hurts and what doesn't work. Some of these problems may reflect changes in the microflora. In addition, digestive function can be affected by other medical difficulties. For example, constipation, diarrhoea and heartburn are common side effects of medications.

At least five studies, some unpublished, have found that probiotic bacteria can relieve constipation in older adults, according to a review article that appeared in the *Postgraduate Medical Journal* in 2004. Moreover, we already know that a fibre-rich diet – recommended in this book for its prebiotic value – counters constipation.

Age-related changes in the microflora make us more susceptible to *Clostridium difficile*, which causes diarrhoea. This bacterium is normally present in our GI tract, but its numbers are kept in check by friendly bacteria. Probiotics such as *Lactobacillus rhamnosus* GG and *Saccharomyces boulardii* lyo have proven very effective at treating diarrhoea caused by *C. difficile*. Though their ability to *prevent* the problem is not yet proven, it seems probable that they'd be useful for that as well.

➤ PROBIOTICS AND THE MENOPAUSE ◀

As women go through the menopause, their vaginal microflora changes. The population of *E. coli* increases, while the probiotic *Lactobacilli* decline. The reason isn't clear, but we assume that hormonal changes are involved. For example, we know that lower oestrogen levels alter the surface of the vaginal tract. One possibility is that these oestrogen-related changes make the environment less hospitable to *Lactobacilli* – and if they have a harder time growing on the vaginal lining, other microbes will crowd them out. This theory is supported by the fact that postmenopausal women who take hormone replacement therapy have higher levels of *Lactobacilli* than those who don't.

At least in part because of changes in their microflora, women become more vulnerable to vaginal infections after the menopause. This is yet another reason to consume probiotics, as Chapter 8 will explain.

Preventing Urinary Tract Infections

Starting in midlife, men and women are vulnerable to urinary tract infections. Blame it on age-related changes in the microflora plus prostate problems for men and the menopause for women. Chapter 8 summarises evidence that probiotics are useful for treating and preventing these conditions.

Toning the Immune System

Have you ever wondered why, when the flu vaccine is in short supply, people over 65 are given higher priority than other adults? That's because our immune system needs more support as we age. Like other systems of the body, it simply doesn't function as well as it did when we were younger.

Several studies have shown that a variety of probiotic regimens can improve white blood cell counts in older people. Does that translate into better health? Apparently so. Italian investigators recruited adults over the age of 60 for a study to see if probiotics could reduce the impact of winter infections. Half of the participants were assigned at random to receive a milk drink supplemented with *Lactobacillus bulgaricus, Streptococcus thermophilus* and *L. casei* DN-114 001; the rest drank a similar beverage without the probiotics. Neither group was free of respiratory and gastrointestinal infections, but those who received probiotics had significantly shorter illnesses with less fever. The results were published in the *Journal of Nutrition, Health and Aging* in 2003.

There's much more to learn about ageing, the microflora and probiotics. But as a middle-aged adult, I'm encouraged by what we know already. Just as physical exercise can delay the ageing of our muscles, bones and cardiovascular system, it appears that probiotics help us to maintain a more youthful microflora, with a wide range of benefits for health.

WHAT ABOUT FIDO AND FLUFFY?

Research suggests that companion animals benefit just as much from probiotics as we do. So it's not surprising that some pet food manufacturers are beginning to offer foods that incorporate probiotics and prebiotics. Probiotic supplements are also available for cats and dogs. Should you give these products to your pets? And what about yoghurt or other products intended for human consumption?

Ask your vet. Many veterinarians – including the one who cares for my pets – are accumulating favourable experiences with probiotics.

CHAPTER SIX

Digestive Diseases

The digestive system is a miracle worker. It can take a tuna mayonnaise sandwich, convert it into fuel for a quick football match, and transform any leftovers into fat molecules to be stored for future energy needs. Unfortunately, a lot can go wrong in the process. Millions of patients in the United Kingdom suffer from digestive diseases. Each year, problems with the digestive tract prompt millions of doctor visits and trips to hospital. And that's just the people whose problems are severe enough to warrant professional attention. Many millions more end up at their local chemist, where shelves are stocked with products that promise relief for wind, indigestion, diarrhoea or constipation.

A well-balanced gut microflora – one with a strong population of probiotic bacteria – goes a long way towards ensuring healthy functioning of the digestive tract. We're beginning to learn that many gastrointestinal problems, including some previously attributed to other causes, in fact originate in microflora imbalances or in improper immune responses. These new insights have prompted a flood of scientific research about possible therapeutic roles for probiotics. Though this research is still at an early stage, preliminary findings are encouraging. Probiotics offer the hope of treatments that are not only effective, but also inexpensive and free of the harmful side effects that conventional drugs often cause.

INFLAMMATORY BOWEL DISEASE

When your gut develops damage and inflammation, you're in trouble. That's what happens in inflammatory bowel disease (IBD) – chronic inflammatory conditions of the large and small intestines. The symptoms are terrible: debilitating diarrhoea, abdominal pain and exhaustion – and the misery is difficult to cure. After all, a doctor can't clean and bandage the intestines, nor can they be kept sterile. Happily, probiotics show great promise for dealing with the problem.

The two most common forms of IBD are ulcerative colitis (which affects the lining of the large intestine and the rectum) and Crohn's disease (which can occur anywhere in the digestive tract). About 140,000 people in the United Kingdom suffer from IBD or about 1 in every 400 people. The condition can affect anyone, from children to the elderly, but it usually begins before the age of 30.

How IBD Starts

Inflammatory bowel disease is an autoimmune condition. It starts when the immune system mistakes normal digestive tract bacteria for dangerous microbes and attacks them. As a result, blood flows to the area and an inflammatory process begins. Helper T cells and pagocytes – the specialised white blood cells you read about in Chapter 4 – release chemicals designed to destroy microbial enemies. But in IBD, they also damage the intestinal lining; sometimes this creates ulcers (open sores).

The damage amplifies the call for blood, producing more inflammation and more damage to the bowel. The problem is exacerbated if, as often happens, the normal bacteria they're targeting remain in the microflora or are constantly reintroduced. No matter how much tissue is destroyed, the immune system persists in trying to eliminate what it perceives as a microbial invader.

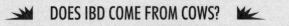

DOES IBD COME FROM COWS?

One theory is that bacteria transmitted from cows to humans may initiate IBD. A cattle ailment called Johne's disease appears to be identical to Crohn's disease in humans. The symptoms are the same; the appearances of affected cow and human intestines are the same.

Johne's disease is caused by *Mycobacterium avium* ssp *paratuberculosis* (abbreviated MAP). Direct contact with infected cows isn't required to transmit MAP to humans, because the bacteria are present in their milk and meat. Though MAP can be killed by ultrapasteurisation (pasteurisation at extra-high temperature), it survives both standard pasteurisation and ordinary cooking.

Some experts believe that MAP causes Crohn's disease in humans. However, others point out that in areas where MAP exposure is high, such as rural areas and on farms, Crohn's disease is actually less common than in urban areas. Research is under way to address the question.

It's not yet clear what triggers this perverse immune response. Nor do we understand why the regulatory T cells, which normally counter unnecessary inflammation, fail to respond appropriately in IBD. The condition runs in families, so a genetic component may be involved. Environmental factors also appear to play a role: IBD occurs most often in people who live in cities and in developed countries.

Symptoms

The symptoms of ulcerative colitis and Crohn's disease are so similar that it's often difficult to differentiate the two without direct examination of the intestinal tract. As inflammation and ulcers develop, patients experience frequent and sometimes bloody diarrhoea, as well as severe abdominal pain and cramping. Secondary problems may occur, such as fatigue, drastic weight loss and malnutrition and anaemia resulting from loss of blood. Even worse are possible complications, including intestinal blockage, which is caused by swelling and scarring of the intestinal walls.

Though the condition is chronic, the course of the disease typically involves acute flare-ups followed by periods of remission. An IBD flare-up is like having a bad intestinal virus that simply won't go away. On top of the pain and disability, people with active ulcerative colitis or Crohn's disease are forced to plan their lives around having quick access to a toilet. Jobs and relationships suffer. Depression often accompanies IBD – and it isn't simply an emotional response to pain and disability. Along with inflammation, the immune system produces chemicals that act on the parts of the brain that affect mood.

Conventional Treatments for Inflammatory Bowel Disease

Various medical treatments are used to address the symptoms and underlying causes of IBD. But IBD is a chronic condition. Even if an acute flare-up is resolved, the problem can return. Therefore the medications described below are prescribed to prevent new attacks as well as for treatment. These drugs must be taken for a lifetime, and unfortunately, most have adverse side effects.

Anti-Inflammatory Drugs

The inflammation of IBD often can be brought under control with anti-inflammatory drugs, such as prednisone, a corticosteroid. These powerful drugs can bring relief in a matter of days – but they come with potentially disastrous consequences. If used for a prolonged period, corticosteroids can cause Cushing's syndrome, which produces significant effects on health and appearance. People with Cushing's syndrome retain water and gain weight. Their faces become round and puffy, with associated swelling in the neck, upper back and abdomen. Women may develop excess facial and body hair. Acne and other skin problems are common. Other side effects include muscle weakness in the arms and legs, fragile bones, high blood sugar, fatigue and mood swings. Because of these considerable risks, corticosteroids are not recommended for long-term use.

Antibiotics

Antibiotics help to relieve IBD because they eliminate the intestinal microbes against which the immune system is reacting. However, additional medication usually is required to address inflammation. Moreover, symptoms often return in full force after antibiotics are discontinued: the intestinal microflora repopulates and the immune system again launches its unnecessary attack against them.

Surgery

Damage to the intestinal tract from IBD is often so extensive that medication can't repair or relieve it. An estimated 25 to 40 per cent of those with ulcerative colitis, and up to 75 per cent of those with Crohn's disease, eventually require surgical treatment. Surgery may be used to widen blocked areas of the intestines or to excise diseased portions. Sometimes symptoms are so extensive and severe that the only solution is to remove the entire colon and rectum, despite the drastic lifestyle changes required when body wastes must be collected by artificial replacements.

The Role of Probiotics

The cruel dilemma that people with IBD face is how to balance the suffering caused by the disease against that associated with treatment. These drawbacks make the potential of probiotics even more attractive.

We know that inflammation-fighting regulatory T cells are deficient in the intestines of IBD patients. As you'll recall from Chapter 4, probiotics can stimulate production of regulatory T cells. But studies show that people with inflammatory bowel disease have lower levels of probiotics in their intestinal microflora than do healthy individuals. Moreover, among IBD patients, those with the active disease have fewer probiotics than those in remission. All this suggests that boosting these beneficial microbes could be a powerful yet safe way to prevent and treat the condition.

Preventing IBD with Probiotics

Preliminary findings from animal studies suggest that a wide range of probiotic bacteria can protect against IBD. These investigations use laboratory rats and mice that stack the odds in favour of getting the disease. Some of the animals have been genetically altered so that their immune system doesn't function properly; as a result, they spontaneously develop IBD a few months after birth.

In other experiments, the rats or mice are treated with chemicals that irritate the intestinal tract.

Even in these animals, which are especially vulnerable to IBD, a variety of probiotic therapies can prevent it. The probiotics used successfully include *Lactobacillus reuteri*, *L. plantarum* 299v and *L. rhamnosus* GG. Another effective preventive treatment is a commercial product called VSL#3, which blends eight probiotic bacteria, including species of *Bifidobacterium* and *Lactobacillus*, as well as a probiotic species of *Streptococcus*.

Treating IBD with Probiotics

An exciting pilot study of human patients, published in 2003 in the *European Journal of Gastroenterology and Hepatology*, showed that a probiotic yeast, *Saccharomyces boulardii*, could be used instead of steroids to decrease intestinal inflammation in people with ulcerative colitis. Antibiotics are often used in combination with steroids to counter IBD. Investigators recruited patients who were taking antibiotics, but who couldn't use steroids because of terrible side effects that included the development of diabetes, water retention, skin rashes and persistent indigestion.

At the start of the study, patients were given physical examinations as well as blood tests to check for inflammation. Then for four weeks they took three capsules daily of the probiotic, along with prescribed antibiotics. Twenty-four patients completed this treatment. At the end, they were re-examined and questioned about their symptoms. Seventeen of them (71 per cent) showed significant improvement. This evaluation was based not only on their subjective reports, but also on blood tests for inflammation and direct examination of the large intestine with a viewing instrument called a sigmoidoscope. Another important result was that not one of these patients – all of whom had experienced significant medical problems when taking steroids – reported side effects from the probiotic supplement.

Though these and other findings about ulcerative colitis are very encouraging, we currently have less evidence that probiotics are effective in treating Crohn's disease. Some pilot studies show benefits from *Saccharomyces boulardii*, *E. coli* Nissle 1917 and *Lactobacillus rhamnosus* GG. But other preliminary investigations failed to confirm these findings. Nevertheless, medical researchers remain extremely enthusiastic about probiotics as a potential therapy for Crohn's disease, too.

TREATING ILEAL POUCHITIS WITH PROBIOTICS

People with chronic ulcerative colitis sometimes have such severe symptoms that their entire colon and rectum is removed. One option in this situation is to collect wastes in an external bag that's attached to the abdomen. As an alternative, some patients undergo complex surgery to create an internal rectum substitute from the ileum, the lowest part of the small intestine. This is called an ileal pouch.

While this solution has obvious advantages, one disadvantage is that inflammatory responses sometimes develop around the pouch – a condition called ileal pouchitis. Ironically, the symptoms resemble those of ulcerative colitis. Antibiotics can often clear up the problem, but it's likely to return. Also, about 10 per cent of patients with recurring pouchitis don't respond to antibiotics.

Two carefully conducted trials have shown that the probiotic blend VSL#3 can dramatically reduce the chances that pouchitis will recur after treatment. In one study, 85 per cent of those who took VSL#3 were free of symptoms for nine months; in contrast, only 6 per cent of those in the control group escaped a relapse. The other study had similar findings. VSL#3 has also been found effective in preventing IBD in animal studies. The search is on for probiotic therapies that could treat pouchitis while the infection is still active.

Dr John Kao, an National Institutes of Health-funded gastroenterology researcher at the University of Michigan Medical School, comments, 'Probiotics hold great promise as a new therapy that we can use with other interventions to effectively treat inflammatory bowel diseases, such as ulcerative colitis and Crohn's disease. The challenge at the moment is identifying the optimal type and dose of probiotic to use.' Accordingly, additional controlled trials are under way with a variety of probiotics to determine which ones will be most effective in treating flare-ups or preventing relapses during remission.

IRRITABLE BOWEL SYNDROME

Most people have a feeling of fullness after consuming a large meal. But a person with irritable bowel syndrome (IBS) often develops uncomfortable bloating and cramping. Other common symptoms are similar to those of inflammatory bowel disease, though usually less severe: abdominal pain, wind and diarrhoea or constipation. The bowel isn't damaged, as it is in IBD. Rather, the nerves and muscles of the intestines overreact to normal stimulation. The problem may be continuous, or the patient may experience flare-ups followed by periods of remission.

According to BUPA, IBS is one of the most common disorders of the digestive tract, and about one-fifth of people in the UK experience symptoms. The underlying cause of IBS is still a matter of speculation. Recently, attention has focused on two intriguing possibilities – one involving gut microbes and the other involving inflammation – that raise the hope that probiotics could help.

Small Intestinal Bacterial Overgrowth (SIBO): A Possible Cause of IBS

The most common symptom of IBS is excess wind build-up in the small intestine after a meal. This stretches the small intestine, causing the bloating and pain that characterise the condition. Because many different foods produce the same problem, most medical scientists have assumed that IBS is not caused by an allergy or intolerance towards a specific food. Instead, some hypothesise, the reason could be a condition called small intestinal bacterial overgrowth (SIBO), in which the microflora of the large intestine invades the small intestine. If this is indeed the cause, probiotics may offer the solution.

Explaining the Symptoms

Normally, different types of bacteria live in the small and large intestines and they have different jobs to do. One important difference involves digestion of the carbohydrates in our food. Most of these carbohydrates are absorbed in the small intestine. But one type of complex carbohydrate – dietary fibre – passes through the small intestine; it's not broken down until it reaches the large intestine. The microbes of the small intestine don't produce much wind when they process other forms of carbohydrate. But as people who've introduced high-fibre foods to their diet can attest, when the microflora of the large intestine digests fibre, wind is often a by-product. In the large intestine, wind isn't a serious problem. Other resident microbes absorb most of it, and since the large intestine is adjacent to the rectum and anus, any excess is easily released as flatulence.

Some scientists have proposed that SIBO could explain the symptoms of IBS. If wind-producing microbes from the large intestine take up residence in the small intestine, they may process fibre there instead of letting it pass through undigested, as microbes native to the small intestine would do. The resulting wind is not readily absorbed by other microbes and has no easy exit. So the wind distends the small intestine, producing bloating and discomfort.

A microbial explanation for IBS also could account for the otherwise puzzling discrepancy in symptoms found in people with the condition: some suffer from constipation, while others have diarrhoea. Symptoms could vary depending on the particular microbes that have overgrown. (Despite the term 'small intestinal *bacterial* overgrowth', overgrowth of the yeast *Candida albicans* – normally an inhabitant of the large intestine – may also be involved in SIBO.)

Causes

Normally, three factors prevent bacteria in the large intestine from overgrowing into the small intestine:

• **Acids in the small intestine:** During digestion, the contents of the stomach – including all the acid and digestive enzymes – empty into the small intestine. This environment is great for breaking down food but harsh for bacterial survival.
• **Peristalsis:** The contractions that move the contents of the digestive tract create what is normally a one-way street from the oesophagus to the anus. That makes it difficult for bacteria from the large intestine to move in the opposite direction.
• **Microbial competition:** Chemicals produced by the normal microflora of the small intestine help to prevent microflora from the large intestine from taking over.

Anything that disrupts these influences can contribute to SIBO. This includes many common medications. For example, a person who frequently takes antacids to neutralise stomach acids is also making the small intestine less acidic – and therefore more vulnerable to bacterial overgrowth. Taking a medication that decreases peristalsis (as some antidepressants do) also removes a natural protection against SIBO. How can you tell that a drug might decrease peristalsis? Look for constipation on the list of possible side effects. Antibiotics, which may disrupt the protective microflora of the small intestine, also can enable overgrowth.

⚡ DIAGNOSING SIBO ⚡

The ideal way to diagnose SIBO (small intestinal bacterial overgrowth) would be to extract a microflora sample from the small intestine and then analyse the bacteria it contains. But that would require snaking an instrument down the throat, through the stomach and into the gut, a process that's invasive, risky and expensive – not to mention uncomfortable. Instead, doctors use a breath test that detects hydrogen.

After an eight-to-twelve-hour fast to clear the digestive tract, the patient consumes a small amount of a man-made sugar called lactulose that's not digested by bacteria that normally live in the small intestine, but that can be broken down by bacteria of the large intestine. As these bacteria digest the lactulose, they release hydrogen gas, which is absorbed by blood vessels in the walls of the large intestine. The blood-stream carries the hydrogen to the lungs, where it's transferred to an airway and then exhaled.

During the test, the patient's breath is checked for hydrogen every fifteen minutes. In a healthy person, hydrogen appears once: when the lactulose arrives in the large intestine. But in a person with SIBO, exhaled hydrogen levels usually increase twice – the first time when the lactulose reaches the part of the small intestine where large-intestine bacteria are growing, and then again when the remaining lactulose arrives in the large intestine.

IBS and Inflammation: the 'Stomach Flu' Connection

Until recently, medical experts have assumed that irritable bowel syndrome – unlike inflammatory bowel disease – doesn't involve inflammation. But some researchers are now reconsidering this assumption; they suggest that IBS may involve intestinal inflammation after all.

IBS often develops following a bout of what's popularly known as 'stomach flu' – a misnomer for a disease that is not caused by the influenza virus. The condition, more properly called viral gastroenteritis, is caused by a virus such as norovirus, rotavirus or adenovirus. During an episode of gastroenteritis, the stomach and intestinal linings become inflamed. As with other illnesses, the inflammation normally goes away when the disease is gone. But many studies – based on either blood tests or intestinal tract biopsies – have found that patients who develop IBS after gastroenteritis continue to have low-grade inflammation in their intestinal tract.

The continuing presence of inflammation could help to explain IBS symptoms. Most experts believe that the pain of IBS comes not only from the stretching of the small intestine caused by wind, but also from hypersensitivity of nerves in the intestinal tract. When tissue is chronically inflamed, nerves in that tissue become hypersensitive. In addition, there could be a link between inflammation and small intestinal bacterial overgrowth. Chemicals released by white blood cells during low-level inflammation of the intestinal tract can affect the nerves and muscles in a way that decreases peristalsis – a factor in SIBO.

Treating IBS with Probiotics

Standard treatments for IBS have focused on relieving symptoms. Recommended measures include dietary changes, stress reduction and medications to address pain, constipation, diarrhoea, and other symptoms. But if it turns out that inflammation and small intestinal bacterial overgrowth are involved in IBS, probiotics would be an ideal therapy. Probiotics stimulate regulatory T cell responses, which decrease inflammation. They also produce chemicals that control bacterial overgrowth. At the same time, they're safe for long-term use.

Findings from clinical trials suggest that certain probiotics can reduce IBS symptoms. For example, Irish investigators recruited 77 patients with IBS to assess the effectiveness of two probiotic strains in treating the condition. Patients were divided into three groups: the first group received a daily dose of a probiotic, *Lactobacillus salivarius* UCC4331, delivered in a malted milk drink; the second drank the same beverage but with a different probiotic, *Bifidobacterium infantis* 35624; and the third group was given a placebo – plain malted milk. None of the patients knew which version they were drinking. For four weeks before they began drinking the malted milk, and then during the next eight weeks, participants recorded their symptoms. They were told not to take any medications such as laxatives, anti-diarrhoeal agents, antibiotics or commercially available probiotic preparations.

Patients who drank the beverage containing *Bifidobacterium infantis* 35624 showed significant improvement in abdominal pain, bloating and regularity of bowel movements. However, no benefit over the placebo was seen in those who received *Lactobacillus salivarius* UCC4331. The findings, which were published in 2005 in the journal *Gastroenterology*, underscore the importance of testing a variety of probiotics when developing treatments.

⚡ A CASE HISTORY ⚡

For Mordechai Eliezer Smith, age 58, a certain type of cramping gives the warning. 'It hits mid-abdomen and goes straight down, like a rising peristaltic wave. It hits once, and I know that it's going to repeat.' Mordechai has learnt from experience that he desperately needs to be in the toilet when that happens.

Six years ago, he was diagnosed with irritable bowel syndrome by Dr David Rubin, a University of Chicago gastro-enterologist. But the difficulties began before that. Recalls Mordechai, 'It made me a miserable person. I wouldn't know if it was going to be five hours or five minutes before I'd have to run to the bathroom again. Sometimes the pain was excruciating and the cramping was unbearable. This limited my going out with people. A few times the pain was so terrible that I would have to lie in bed. Any movement I made would exacerbate the pain.'

'We've been up and down in managing his condition,' says Dr Rubin. Two years ago, he gave Mordechai samples of the probiotic yeast *Saccharomyces boulardii*. Mordechai says, 'The difference became apparent in four or five days. I was really regular. It was amazing. I didn't know it was possible.'

Dr Rubin comments, 'I've used this probiotic yeast in a few patients who have diarrhoea-predominant irritable bowel syndrome. Mordechai is one of the most dramatic examples of success. There's so much we don't understand about what causes an irritable bowel. But there's reason to think that balancing flora in the gut is effective.'

PEPTIC ULCERS

According to BUPA's Health Information Team, up to one in ten Britons will develop a peptic ulcer at some time in his or her life. A peptic ulcer is a sore or hole in the lining of the stomach (gastric ulcer) or at the beginning of the small intestine (duodenal ulcer). This damage produces abdominal pain (the most common symptom) and also nausea, bloating, burping, poor appetite and fatigue. About two decades ago, researchers demonstrated that *Helicobacter pylori* bacteria are responsible for most ulcers. However, long-term use of aspirin and other non-steroidal anti-inflammatory drugs (NSAIDs) can cause similar problems.

Why Ulcers Develop

The mere presence of *Helicobacter pylori* in the stomach is not enough to cause ulcers. About 40 per cent of British people carry the bacteria – yet most don't develop the problem. Thus it's clear that other factors contribute. We know that the immune system is involved, because ulcers result from an inflammatory response against *H. pylori*. But not everyone responds to the presence of these bacteria with inflammation. For reasons we don't under-stand, some people can live with them, as if they were normal members of the stomach microflora – in other words, their immune system tolerates the bacteria.

Can Probiotics Prevent Ulcers?

Since high levels of *Helicobacter pylori* are required to develop an ulcer, scientists have wondered if probiotics might reduce the risk by limiting growth of the bacteria. Laboratory experiments have established that numerous strains of *Lactobacillus* – including *L. acidophilus, L. johnsonii L. salivarius* and *L. casei* – can indeed slow the growth of *H. pylori* in a Petri dish, and sometimes even kill it.

⟫ PROVING THAT BACTERIA CAUSE ULCERS ⟪

In the early 1980s, two Australian doctors, J Robin Warren and Barry J Marshall, isolated *Helicobacter pylori* from the stomachs of ulcer patients. But their suggestion that these bacteria actually caused the ulcers was met with general disbelief for more than a decade. The standard explanation for ulcers at the time was that they resulted from excess stomach acid that was produced by emotional stress and improper diet. A bacterial cause seemed outlandish, because medical experts believed that bacteria couldn't survive in the acidic environment of the stomach.

In frustration, Dr Marshall decided to prove the connection by infecting himself. After undergoing a preliminary examination to demonstrate that his stomach was healthy, he drank a pure culture of the bacteria. Five days later he developed severe gastrointestinal symptoms from gastritis, an inflammation of the stomach that is associated with ulcers.

Subsequent research showed that ulcers could be permanently cured with antibiotics that completely eradicated *H. pylori*. Previous ulcer treatments had provided only temporary relief. The new explanation and therapy for ulcers gradually gained acceptance. In 2005, Dr Warren and Dr Marshall shared a Nobel Prize for their discovery.

Deliberately infecting people with *Helicobacter* would raise ethical concerns, so researchers have used laboratory animals to further explore the use of probiotics to prevent ulcers. Since *Lactobacillus* appears to inhibit *Helicobacter* growth, and the normal microflora of mice contains this probiotic, one animal study used the microbe-free mice I described in Chapter 1. Investigators found that if they fed these mice *Helicobacter*, the bacteria readily grew in their stomachs. But if they first fed the microbe-free mice *Lactobacillus salivarius* for a few days, and then tried to introduce *Helicobacter*, the mice were completely protected from the infection. In a follow-up experiment – this time with mice that were already infected with *Helicobacter* – the scientists showed that feeding the mice *Lactobacillus* reduced the presence of *Helicobacter* by more than 99 per cent.

A 2004 study in the *American Journal of Clinical Nutrition* suggests that probiotics are also effective against *H. pylori* in humans who carry the bacteria. Investigators recruited 70 adults who tested positive for *H. pylori*, but who had no symptoms of ulcers. For a six-week period, 59 of the volunteers consumed two daily portions of yoghurt that contained two probiotics: *Lactobacillus acidophilus* La5 and *Bifidobacterium lactis* Bb12. The other 11 volunteers, the control group, drank an equal volume of ordinary milk twice a day. Two weeks after the experiment ended, *Helicobacter* levels were reassessed in all subjects. Those who had consumed probiotic-containing yoghurt had significantly lowered their levels of *H. pylori*; no such benefit was found in the control group.

Interestingly, an additional check-up, performed more than two months after the volunteers had stopped eating the yoghurt, found that *H. pylori* had usually increased again. In other words, probiotics may not eliminate the bacteria that can cause ulcers, but they appear effective at keeping levels low – thereby preventing the damage these bacteria can cause.

Treating Ulcers and Reducing 'Triple Therapy' Side Effects with Probiotics

The standard current treatment for those suffering from peptic ulcers is called 'triple therapy', because it involves a combination of two antibiotics to kill *H. pylori*, plus a third medication to either decrease acid production in the stomach or to protect the stomach from the acids. According to the National Institutes of Health, this treatment is effective in more than 90 per cent of adult patients: it relieves ulcer symptoms, kills the bacteria and prevents ulcer recurrence. In children, the success rate is lower, around 60 per cent. Unfortunately, triple therapy may cause unpleasant side effects, including nausea, diarrhoea, abdominal pain, taste disturbances, headaches and body aches.

Research is currently under way to see if probiotics can increase the effectiveness of triple therapy, particularly in children. There's also hope that probiotics might reduce treatment side effects. Furthermore, if probiotics could replace one or both of the antibiotics used to treat ulcers, this would reduce the risk of *Helicobacter* developing antibiotic resistance. So far, published studies are very encouraging.

For example, Czech investigators studied 86 children who were taking triple therapy for ulcer symptoms. Thirty-nine of the children also received Actimel, the popular milk product that contains the probiotic *Lactobacillus casei* DN-114 001. The remaining children drank the same quantity of regular milk. Neither the patients nor the doctors knew whether the patient was receiving the probiotic in addition to triple therapy.

Four weeks after treatment, the children were re-examined. *Helicobacter* had been eliminated in 60 per cent of the patients receiving triple therapy plus plain milk – a typical response for children given triple therapy alone. However, *Helicobacter* was eliminated in 90 per cent of those whose triple therapy was supplemented by Actimel – a dramatically improved result achieved at low cost and no risk, thanks to probiotics.

Equally strong results have come from research focused on using probiotics to prevent the side effects of triple therapy. Numerous studies have shown that probiotics – including *Lactobacillus rhamnosus* GG, *Saccharomyces boulardii*, mixed *Lactobacillus* species and various strains of *Bifidobacterium* – significantly reduce the unwanted symptoms that normally accompany this treatment.

VIRAL GASTROENTERITIS

Viral gastroenteritis – popularly (but mistakenly) known as 'stomach flu' – is a common illness, familiar to most of us. The major symptoms are diarrhoea and vomiting, but the illness can also include fever, headache, chills and abdominal pain. Most adults recover after a day or two (though, as I mentioned earlier in this chapter, bouts of viral gastroenteritis have been associated with the development of irritable bowel syndrome). But viral gastroenteritis is potentially more serious for children, especially those under the age of 2, because symptoms can last for up to eight days. This can lead to dehydration, which may become life-threatening if the child doesn't drink sufficient fluids to replenish those lost through diarrhoea and vomiting.

The disease is highly contagious. The viruses most often responsible – rotavirus and norovirus – can be transmitted directly from a person who's infected. But it's enough to come into contact with utensils that such a person has handled. Moreover, someone who has recovered from viral gastroenteritis can still spread the infection for a week after their symptoms are gone. These characteristics help to explain why outbreaks often occur in situations where infected food handlers serve large numbers of people, such as cruise ships, restaurants, resorts, and university halls of residence.

The standard therapy for viral gastroenteritis involves drinking plenty of fluids and eating easy-to-digest foods. Electrolyte drinks, which replace essential salts as well as fluids, are also recommended to counter the dehydrating effects of vomiting and diarrhoea. Doctors and medical researchers have wondered whether probiotics might be helpful as well, especially in young children. Several clinical trials suggest that they are.

For instance, investigators at several European medical centres studied a total of 287 children, aged 1 month to 3 years, all of whom had been hospitalised for diarrhoea. One group (140 children) was given a standard electrolyte solution for rehydration, while the remaining children received the same solution with *Lactobacillus rhamnosus* GG added. Neither the parents nor the doctors knew which solution contained probiotics.

On average, the duration of the diarrhoea was reduced by an impressive 13 hours – from 71 hours to 58 hours – in the group receiving probiotics. Probiotic treatment was especially effective for diarrhoea caused by rotavirus, reducing the duration of this dangerous symptom by almost a day. The children who received probiotics had shorter hospital stays, on average, than those of children who received the standard rehydration therapy. These results were published in 2000 in the *Journal of Pediatric Gastroenterology and Nutrition*. Other studies have confirmed the efficacy of *L. rhamnosus* GG and demonstrated that *L. rhamnosus* 19070-2 and *L. reuteri* DSM 12246 also reduce the length and severity of viral gastroenteritis in children.

ANTIBIOTIC-ASSOCIATED DIARRHOEA

Diarrhoea is a common side effect of antibiotics. That's not surprising. These drugs destroy not only their target germs, but also probiotic bacteria. As a result, certain diarrhoea-causing microbes, which are normally kept at harmless levels, can proliferate. The problem is usually no more than a nuisance: the patient takes his or her favourite over-the-counter remedy to tame the symptoms, and the situation resolves when the course of antibiotics is over. But one particular form of antibiotic-associated diarrhoea, caused by the bacterium *Clostridium difficile*, can turn serious and even deadly.

Have you ever heard the term 'nosocomial infection'? The word 'nosocomial' comes from the Greek *nosokomeion*, meaning 'hospital'. So it's a fancy way of saying, 'You got this infection in the hospital.' *C. difficile* diarrhoea is usually a nosocomial infection,

➤➤ IN THE SERVICE OF SCIENCE ➤➤

Most people don't look forward to a bout of antibiotic associated diarrhoea. But for Vincent B Young, MD, PhD, an infectious disease specialist at Michigan State University, it represented an opportunity. A broad-spectrum antibiotic had been prescribed for his sinusitis. He knew from a prior experience with a similar drug that it would probably cause diarrhoea. This would allow him to collect samples for a study he and an associate were planning. They wanted to document the link between antibiotic administration and changes in the gut microflora.

Two years earlier, Dr Young had been hospitalised for an abscess in his throat and given broad-spectrum antibiotics. He recalls: 'I developed miserable diarrhoea.' His response was to eat yoghurt. Someone on the medical staff commented that yoghurt would be soothing for his throat. But Dr Young says, 'I wasn't thinking of that. I was thinking of replenishing everything the antibiotics wiped out. The diarrhoea was under control in a day and a half.'

Soon after Dr Young started taking the antibiotic prescribed for his sinusitis, the predicted diarrhoea began. To avoid interfering with data collection for his article, he refrained from eating yoghurt. 'This time,' he reports, 'it took five or six days for things to settle down.' His co-authored research report appeared in the *Journal of Clinical Microbiology* in 2004. It provided an analysis of the specific changes in gastrointestinal bacteria that can lead to antibiotic-associated diarrhoea.

acquired by individuals who are vulnerable in two ways: they're in hospital with other ill people and their resistance to the bacterium is compromised by taking antibiotics. *C. difficile* easily travels from one patient to another when toilets and other surfaces become contaminated, even if the medical staff is diligent about washing their hands. An infection can lead to severe dehydration and a form of colitis that's life-threatening.

According to a 2006 review article in the *American Journal of Gastroenterology,* more than two dozen carefully controlled studies have shown that certain probiotics – *Saccharomyces boulardii, Lactobacillus rhamnosus* GG and various probiotic mixtures – significantly reduced the development of antibiotic-associated diarrhoea. Only S. *boulardii* (a probiotic yeast) was effective against C. *difficile* infection. In Chapter 11, I'll give you detailed information, derived from this research, about preventing and treating antibiotic-associated diarrhoea with probiotics.

TRAVELLERS' DIARRHOEA

The problem usually begins abruptly. In addition to diarrhoea and cramps, a victim of travellers' diarrhoea might experience nausea, vomiting, fever and a sense of malaise. Most cases are not life-threatening; symptoms disappear within a week, even without treatment. But who wants to waste precious holiday time in the toilet? Also, this illness – like all types of diarrhoea – can be dangerous for infants, the elderly, and people with compromised immune systems.

According to the Centers for Disease Control and Prevention, each year an estimated 10 million people, or 20 to 50 per cent of international travellers, come down with diarrhoea either during or shortly after their trip. Typically, a traveller develops symptoms after eating food or drinking water that is contaminated with microbes – bacteria, viruses or parasites – of faecal origin. The most common cause is a type of *E. coli* called enterotoxigenic *E. coli*. This bacteria attaches to intestinal cells and releases a toxin that causes cramping and diarrhoea.

Treatment usually involves taking antibiotics along with medication to address the symptoms. Some travellers claim that probiotics help them to prevent travellers' diarrhoea, but research evidence has been mixed. Very likely that's because we haven't yet identified the particular probiotics that are effective. And it could be that what works against the microbial culprits in one part of the world is less useful against different germs elsewhere. There are some suggestions in Chapter 11 (see page 240) for using probiotics to prevent and treat the problem.

◣ WHY TOURISTS CAN'T DRINK THE WATER ◢

When you travel in a foreign country, have you ever wondered why you can't drink the water without risking gastrointestinal distress – yet the people who live there have no such problems? The reason appears to be that their intestinal microflora protects them from developing diarrhoea from the microbes that contaminate water. However, if natives move away for a long period of time, their microflora changes. Should they return for a visit, they have the same risk of developing 'tourists' disease' as any other traveller.

✸ PROBIOTICS – FOR CHICKENS! ✸

According to the Centers for Disease Control and Prevention, over a million cases of *salmonella* food poisoning occur each year in the United States, mostly from contaminated chicken eggs. Its symptoms, which can last for up to a week, include diarrhoea, fever and abdominal cramps. People usually recover without treatment. But *salmonella* can be fatal to the very young, the very old and those with impaired immune systems.

New strains of *salmonella* can infect the ovaries of hens without causing symptoms of the disease. As a result, eggs may be contaminated even if they look clean and come from apparently healthy chickens. If such eggs are eaten raw or are not cooked properly, food poisoning can result. The 'Lion Quality Mark' on British eggs indicates that they come from hens vaccinated against *salmonella*. The mark is found on more than 80 per cent of eggs in the UK market.

Preliminary evidence suggests that probiotics can help to prevent *salmonella* infection where it starts – in chickens. In one study, researchers included the probiotic *Lactobacillus salivarius* CTC2197 in the feed and drinking water of one group of chickens; a control group received regular feed and drinking water. All the birds were infected with *salmonella* by directly introducing it into their stomachs. Three weeks later, the chickens were examined. Those given regular feed and drinking water showed evidence of *salmonella* growing within them – but the chickens that received the probiotic were *salmonella*-free.

As this chapter detailed, clinical trials have demonstrated the promise of probiotics for treating major digestive disorders. Also exciting is the potential of probiotics to prevent gastrointestinal problems, from debilitating conditions like inflammatory bowel disease to the minor difficulties that all of us experience occasionally, like temporary irregularity.

Medical scientists are working on probiotic therapies that one day will supplement and perhaps even replace other treatments for some digestive tract diseases. But in the meantime, safe and healthy probiotic foods are available at the supermarket. We can start using them today to maximise our gastrointestinal health now – and to help reduce our chances of developing these diseases in the future.

CHAPTER SEVEN

Allergic Diseases

Allergic reactions are hardly new. Hippocrates and other physicians from history described them in their writings. But allergies were a minor disease until about fifty years ago. One nineteenth-century sufferer, the British doctor John Bostock, spent a decade searching for other people with hay fever, and managed to find only two dozen. Today, the pharmaceutical industry advertises hay fever remedies on television, enticing millions of sufferers with the promise of romping through fields of flowers, symptom-free. Imagine how this would astonish Dr Bostock.

Beginning in the 1960s, the rates of hay fever, asthma and other allergies began to rise slowly. The upswing accelerated in the early 1980s. According to a landmark report by the Centers for Disease Control and Prevention in the USA, asthma rates among children aged 5 to 14 jumped by more than 80 per cent between 1980 and 1995. Among people aged 15 to 64, the rise was more than 70 per cent. Over 1 million children and 4 million adults now suffer from asthma in the UK and asthma treatment costs the NHS over £889 million each year.

Other types of allergies followed similar upward trends. According to 2005 statistics from the National Institute of Allergy and Infectious Diseases, more than 50 million Americans have one form of allergy or another. And the United States is not alone. Most of the world's industrialised countries report similar trends in asthma and other allergies. The United Kingdom has the highest asthma rates in the world, followed by Ireland, Australia, New Zealand and Canada.

Though we associate industrial development with improved health, the surprising fact is that rates of allergies and asthma are significantly lower in the undeveloped nations of the world. This difference has led to speculation about the underlying causes of recent increases in the problem – including a deficiency in probiotics.

THE HYGIENE HYPOTHESIS

In 1989, David Strachan, an epidemiologist at the London School of Hygiene and Tropical Medicine, examined the health records of 17,000 British children in search of connections between their allergies and their family life. His analysis showed that the more older siblings they had, the less likely they were to suffer from hay fever. Strachan speculated that the older children were exposing their younger siblings to more viral infections, priming their immune systems so they could better tolerate pollen. He proposed an explanation – later called the 'hygiene hypothesis' – for the rise in hay fever and other allergies. According to the hygiene hypothesis, childhood exposure to microbes, even harmful microbes, is actually beneficial for health, because it helps to protect us from developing allergies.

Another group of researchers, led by John Gerrard at the University Hospital in Saskatoon, Saskatchewan, Canada, had come to a similar conclusion in 1976 after studying the incidence of allergies in white and native (Metis) families living in central Saskatchewan. Gerrard suggested that allergies were 'the price paid by some members of the white community' in exchange for relative freedom from diseases caused by viruses, bacteria and parasites. The hygiene hypothesis offered an explanation for why developing countries, where hygiene standards tend to be lower, have not experienced the surge in allergies seen in developed nations.

Many investigators have explored this provocative idea. For example, subsequent studies found that living on a farm and owning a pet were associated with a lower incidence of allergic diseases. In a major British project, scientists analysed question-naires from more than 10,000 parents of toddlers enrolled in an ongoing study of children's health. Parents were asked questions like 'How often in a normal day are hands washed before meals?' and 'How often does he/she usually have a bath or shower?' From the answers, investigators graded the personal hygiene of each child. Individual scores were compared with health information gathered about the same children several years later. The findings, published in *Archives of Disease in Childhood* in 2002, probably dismayed careful, concerned parents: the higher the hygiene score – in other words, the more washing and wiping the child had received – the more likely the youngster was to develop asthma and allergic dermatitis.

As evidence accumulated in support of the hygiene hypothesis, scientists began to ask a startling question: are we too clean for our own health? In a review article on the subject, immunologists Graham Rook and John Stanford of the University College in

London summarised the answer this way: 'Give us this day our daily germs.'

THE MICROFLORA HYPOTHESIS

At this point you may be wondering if you should stop washing your hands and cleaning your home! So let me put in a few good words about hygiene. Few of us would wish to return to the days of raw sewage in the streets. Exposure to potentially harmful microbes may protect us from allergies, as the hygiene hypothesis suggests. However, these same microbes also can cause diseases far more dangerous than hay fever. Thus, we need to maintain a balance between centuries of progress in public hygiene and reducing the risk of allergies.

As one solution to this dilemma, my colleague Mairi Noverr and I have proposed a revised version of the hygiene hypothesis. We call it the 'microflora hypothesis'. The basic idea (not ours alone, since other scientists have made similar suggestions) is that we do need exposure to microbes to prevent allergies – but that the key microbes for this purpose are the probiotic bacteria in our digestive tract.

Evidence for the microflora hypothesis can be found in studies that compare the gut microflora of individuals who suffer from allergies with that of people who don't. Such research consistently finds that those with allergies have lower levels of probiotic microbes.

In one particularly interesting study, Swedish investigators compared the microbe populations found in stool samples from allergic and non-allergic 2-year-olds. What made this study unusual was that researchers looked at children from both Sweden and Estonia. In general, allergic disease is much more prevalent in Sweden, which is more developed economically. But the study's results showed that living in a country with a high or low rate of allergies was not nearly as important as the bacterial population of a child's digestive tract. Whether Swedish or Estonian, the allergic children were far more likely to have a microflora with decreased levels of probiotic *Lactobacillus* strains and increased levels of *Clostridia* and other potentially harmful bacteria. The results were published in 1999 in *Clinical and Experimental Allergy*.

Public hygiene and exposure to microbes are not the only differences between industrialised and developing countries. Two other relevant factors – both of which affect the gut microflora, as well as the incidence of allergies – are antibiotic use and diet. These are key to the microflora hypothesis.

Antibiotic Use

Antibiotic use is significantly greater in industrialised than in developing countries. Since antibiotics kill probiotic bacteria in the digestive tract, anyone who has taken antibiotics is at risk for insufficient exposure to these essential bacteria. According to the microflora hypothesis, we should see a connection between antibiotic use and subsequent development of allergies. And in fact, numerous studies have found this connection.

One of the largest of such investigations – published in 2002 in the *Journal of Allergy and Clinical Immunology* – was conducted in the United Kingdom, where researchers had access to a medical database that included nearly 30,000 children. Taking antibiotics in the first year of life was associated with an increased incidence of asthma, eczema and hay fever. And the more courses of antibiotics a child had received, the more likely the child was to develop these problems.

Diet

Industrialisation is associated with dietary changes that affect the gut microflora. People in industrialised countries eat significantly more fast food and refined foods, and much less fibre. They're also less likely than people in the developing world to rely on fermentation to preserve food – thus depriving themselves of a ready source of probiotics.

One intriguing study by Swedish researchers focused on children who attend Steiner schools. These schools are based on the teachings of Rudolf Steiner, an early twentieth-century Austrian educator (they're sometimes called Waldorf schools, after the school Steiner established for children of workers at the Waldorf-Astoria cigarette factory in Stuttgart, Germany). Steiner's followers consume a diet that features whole grains, nuts, fruit and vegetables. Investigators found that allergies were significantly less common in children at the Steiner schools compared with children attending ordinary schools nearby. Their report, published in *The Lancet* in 1999, noted that two-thirds of the Steiner school pupils ate fermented vegetables, such as sauerkraut and gherkins.

Implications of the Microflora Hypothesis

The hygiene hypothesis suggests that exposure to microbes, even harmful ones, can protect against allergies. The microflora hypothesis proposes instead that protection comes from exposure to probiotic bacteria in the intestinal microflora. If this theory is correct, then measures to increase the presence of probiotics in the gut should be able to prevent and even treat allergies – without the risk of exposure to harmful microbes. As I'll discuss below, results from numerous animal and human studies are providing strong evidence that probiotics can indeed have these beneficial effects.

ALLERGIC RHINITIS AND HAY FEVER

Allergic rhinitis – an allergy that affects the nose and upper airways – is like a bad cold that never goes away. In a susceptible person, exposure to inhaled allergens – such as animal dander, house dust mites and indoor mould spores – triggers an eruption of symptoms: sneezing, a blocked nose and itchy, red, watery eyes. As if that isn't enough, these problems can lead to a headache, sore throat and difficulties concentrating and sleeping. And on top of everything else, individuals who are vulnerable to respiratory allergies often suffer from asthma and skin rashes, too.

For some, flare-ups are limited to certain times of the year, when particular allergens are prevalent. In such cases, the condition is usually called hay fever or a seasonal allergy. Common seasonal allergens are grass pollens, tree pollens and mould spores. Hay fever affects 15 to 20 per cent of people in the UK.

Conventional Medical Treatments

Imagine being told that you must give up a beloved family pet or that you must remain indoors for months at a time. But 'avoid allergens' is the standard advice given to people with allergic rhinitis. Obviously, this isn't always practical. For those who can't readily escape their allergy triggers, current treatments for allergic rhinitis focus on symptom relief. But medications aren't trouble-free either.

Antihistamines
Allergic symptoms are triggered when mast cells – white blood cells that live under the skin and on all mucosal surfaces – release a chemical called histamine. This chemical is normally a useful part of the body's inflammatory response: it makes the blood vessels dilate, thereby facilitating the movement of white blood cells to injured or infected tissue. But the release of histamine becomes a problem when inflammation isn't needed, as in an allergic reaction.

Antihistamines, as the name suggests, are drugs that counter the effects of histamine; examples include Clarityn, Zyrtec, Benadryl and many others. Though they can relieve respiratory congestion, they often have undesirable side effects. Sleepiness is a problem with some antihistamines. Indeed, over-the-counter insomnia remedies sometimes use antihistamines to promote drowsiness. Other common problems include gastrointestinal distress, headache, rapid heartbeat and a dry mouth.

Decongestants

Blood vessels in the lining of the nose become dilated during an allergic attack. That's what creates inflammation and congestion. Medications to narrow these blood vessels – such as Beechams, Lemsip, Day Nurse, Sudafed and others – can be administered orally or via nasal sprays or drops. But there are potential downsides. Decongestants can increase blood pressure, because the blood vessels in the nose are not the only ones narrowed by these drugs. And since they're stimulants, they also can cause sleep problems and feelings of nervousness.

Ironically, one common side effect of decongestants is an eventual increase in congestion. This is called the 'rebound effect', and it's most likely to happen to someone who uses this kind of medication for more than a few days – in other words, someone with allergies.

The Option of Probiotics

Early trials of probiotics, administered via both yoghurt and supplements, show significant benefits in relieving allergic rhinitis. Furthermore, they're free of the troubling side effects of traditional medications, which makes them appropriate for long-term use.

Chinese investigators studied the benefits of yoghurt in 80 teenagers and children over the age of 5 who came to a paediatric allergy clinic for treatment. All had suffered from allergic rhinitis for at least a year. They were told to consume one or two servings per day of a yoghurt drink, depending on their size. Twenty children received an ordinary yoghurt drink; the others were given the same beverage enriched with an additional probiotic called *Lactobacillus paracasei* 33. During the study period, the children and their parents were questioned about their symptoms and asked to rate how troublesome their allergies were.

After thirty days, both groups showed improvements. However, the relief from allergic rhinitis symptoms was greater for those who received the drink containing *Lactobacillus paracasei* 33. Particularly encouraging was the fact that no undesirable side effects were caused by this treatment. The results were reported in *Pediatric Allergy and Immunology* in 2004. A subsequent study by another team at the same hospital found similar success with *Lactobacillus paracasei* 33 given as supplements rather than in a drink.

Benefits aren't limited to children. A University of California, Davis, study followed the health of 60 adults in two age ranges: 20 to 40 years old and 50 to 70 years old. Twenty participants were assigned at random to consume a serving of plain yoghurt every day for a year; the yoghurt contained live probiotics. Another twenty also were given plain yoghurt with the same instructions – but this yoghurt had been heat-treated to kill the bacteria. Neither the participants nor the researchers knew which type of yoghurt each person received. A third group of 20, the controls, were asked to refrain from eating yoghurt for a year.

During the study period, subjects filled out weekly questionnaires about their health. Their responses showed a significantly lower level of allergy symptoms for those who consumed yoghurt – with the best results for the group that received yoghurt with live bacteria. Most important, similar benefits were found in both age ranges. These findings were published in the *Journal of Nutrition* in 1999.

ASTHMA

Many people who suffer from allergic rhinitis or hay fever also have asthma, a chronic inflammatory disease of the lungs. It's a savage one-two punch: allergies make it difficult to breathe air *in*; asthma interferes with breathing *out*.

In asthma, swollen, inflamed airways chronically produce excess mucus. The situation becomes even worse during an asthma attack, when the muscles that surround the airways contract, further limiting the flow of air. To get a sense of what that's like, purse your lips and try to breathe in and out through your mouth. Your chest may heave with the effort, but hardly any air is getting through. Of course, you can simply open your mouth and gulp in a deep breath. Asthma isn't so simple. An asthma attack is terrifying, and for good reason. Breathing can become so impaired that the situation is life-threatening. Every six hours one person in Britain dies of an asthma attack.

Asthma has become one of the most common chronic diseases in children, affecting 1.1 million children in the UK, according to Asthma UK. The condition is not confined to children (see box on next page about adult asthma). About 5.2 million British people of all ages suffer from this condition.

Current Approaches to Asthma Management

Current therapies for asthma focus on avoiding triggers. Though asthma always involves chronically inflamed airways, attacks can be triggered in different ways. In people with allergic asthma, attacks result when the immune system responds to an inhaled allergen, such as pollen, mould spores or animal dander. In non-allergic asthma, similar reactions may be caused by cold air, exercise, certain medications (aspirin is one culprit) and cigarette smoke and other air pollution.

⚔ ADULT-ONSET ASTHMA ⚔

There has been a rise of 400,000 in the number of adults with asthma in the UK since the last audit of UK asthma in 2001. Because of concern about asthma in children, it's easy to forget that the disease can start for the first time in adulthood.

Adult-onset asthma is more common in women than it is in men, leading experts to suspect that female hormones may play a role. There's other evidence of a hormonal connection: some women develop adult-onset asthma during pregnancy or when they're going through the menopause. Also, those who take supplemental oestrogen after the menopause are more likely to develop asthma afterwards.

The wheezing and other characteristic symptoms of asthma are the same in adults and children. But the condition often isn't diagnosed as quickly in adults, especially older adults. That's because they're more likely to have other medical problems – such as heart disease or a lung disease like emphysema or bronchitis – with similar symptoms. In addition, adults may mistakenly attribute asthma-related problems, such as breathlessness, to ageing or being out of shape.

Diagnosing asthma and differentiating it from other possible conditions is important, because proper treatment can bring relief. However, treating asthma can be even more challenging for older people than it is for children. Adults are more likely than children to be taking medications for other problems, raising the possibility of adverse drug interactions. Also, adults may have other medical conditions that can be worsened by asthma medication.

Medications, including inhaled drugs that relax the muscles of the airways, provide quick relief if breathing becomes difficult. But the trade-off, as always, is side effects. For severe asthma, inhaled steroids and oral anti-inflammatory medications are used to address the underlying inflammation in the lungs. Among the side effects of asthma inhalers are elevated blood pressure, rapid heartbeat, nervousness and nausea. Long-term use of inhaled steroids may slow a child's growth or cause thinning and bruising of the skin. In addition, there's always a risk of yeast infections in the mouth because the steroids prevent the immune system from controlling yeast growth.

Interest in Probiotics

Research is under way in the United States and also in Finland to determine if probiotics can prevent asthma in children. (See the box on page 147.) This interest is not surprising. Asthma is an inflammatory condition. Normally, the airways don't become inflamed when they're exposed to harmless microbes and temperature changes. But in people with asthma, they do. This suggests that their anti-inflammatory mechanisms aren't working properly. As I explained in Chapter 4, we already know that probiotics can help the immune system to develop regulatory T cells, the white blood cells that travel through the body and turn off inflammation. And studies show that development of asthma correlates very strongly with a decrease in the number of probiotic bacteria in the gut. Put all this together, and it makes perfect sense to hope that probiotics can help to prevent and treat asthma.

In Chapter 1, I described the ground-breaking study that Mairi Noverr and I conducted, which showed that laboratory mice became vulnerable to allergic reactions in their lungs because of changes in their gut microflora. Like humans, mice with respiratory allergies have inflamed lungs – that's what increases their risk of asthma. Currently, my laboratory is performing animal studies to further understand the mechanisms that link asthma and allergies, the immune system and probiotics. We already know that certain changes in the microflora balance decrease the regulatory T cell population and make the animals more vulnerable to respiratory allergies and asthma. But does the microflora produce any other relevant changes in the immune system? We're looking for answers to that question. Also on the agenda is testing a variety of probiotics to see if any can reduce lung inflammation in mice with respiratory allergies.

ECZEMA AND ATOPIC DERMATITIS

Imagine having chronic nettle rash. That's what it's like to suffer from eczema, an intensely uncomfortable skin condition involving inflammation, redness, itching and often blistering. Constant itching provokes scratching, which exacerbates inflammation. The urge to scratch may be so irresistible that the skin breaks, causing bleeding and leading to infections. As you'd guess, eczema may be unsightly and embarrassing. Bad enough if you have skin problems on the limbs or torso – but it's even worse when the face is affected.

The most common form of eczema is atopic dermatitis. The term 'atopic' refers to an allergic response; 'dermatitis' means skin inflammation. In the UK up to one-fifth of children and up to one-twelfth of the adult population have eczema.

Eczema tends to run in families and is not contagious. The problem often begins in infancy and continues through young adulthood. However, adults can be affected, too. In babies, eczema is usually found on the face and scalp. In older children and adults, the condition most often affects the skin in back of the elbows and knees, or the face, neck and upper chest.

CAN PROBIOTICS PREVENT ASTHMA IN CHILDREN?

To answer this question, Dr Michael Cabana, chief of the Division of General Pediatrics at the University of California San Francisco (UCSF) Children's Hospital, is in the process of recruiting nearly 300 newborns. To join this ambitious study, the babies must be healthy and have been born full-term at a normal weight. In addition, they must be at risk for asthma because at least one of their parents has the condition.

Says Dr Cabana, 'Asthma is now one of the most common chronic diseases in children. Here in San Francisco, one child in ten has asthma. We have methods to treat it, but currently there are no known ways to prevent it.'

The UCSF study was inspired by Finnish research (described later in this chapter) showing that eczema could be prevented in infants by giving their mothers supplements during pregnancy. Dr Cabana explains, 'Asthma is related to eczema; they travel together. So it seemed that it would be a natural to study the effect on asthma.'

Half of the infants will be chosen at random to receive a daily supplement of *Lactobacillus* GG during the first six months of their lives; the rest will receive a placebo. The babies will be followed for three years, with regular check-ups starting at the age of one month to look for any early signs of asthma. Such signs include frequent wheezing; wheezing when there's no obvious reason, such as a cold or the flu; frequent runny nose; and eczema.

'A lot of what we do as paediatricians is prevention,' says Dr Cabana. 'It would be a great thing to be able to prevent asthma – and using probiotics could potentially be a safe and effective way to do that.'

Preventing and Treating Eczema

Susceptible individuals develop eczema not only from exposure to skin irritants, but also in response to inhaled allergens or food allergens. As with any allergy, standard medical advice is to avoid the allergens that trigger the problem. But this advice may be nearly impossible to follow. In highly sensitive people, outbreaks may be caused by ubiquitous substances they can't escape: dust, soap or even their own perspiration. Since stress can exacerbate eczema, stress reduction measures also are advised.

The goal of eczema treatment is to relieve itching and inflammation. The skin may be soothed by topical hydrocortisone and other anti-inflammatory ointments, as well as by moisturisers. Another approach involves antihistamines to stop the allergic response that causes eczema. If the skin is broken and becomes infected by bacteria, an antibiotic may be prescribed; this medication may come in the form of an ointment to be applied directly to the skin, or it may be given as a pill or liquid taken orally.

The Promise of Probiotics

Scientific studies show that probiotics can prevent and treat atopic dermatitis. In one very encouraging investigation, which I mentioned briefly in Chapter 1, Finnish doctors recruited 159 pregnant women whose babies were at above-average risk for eczema because of a family history of allergic eczema, allergic rhinitis or asthma.

Volunteers were assigned at random to receive probiotic supplements (*Lactobacillus rhamnosus* GG) or a lookalike placebo; neither the women nor the investigators knew who received which. The mothers-to-be took the capsules for two to four weeks before their due date. After the babies were born, breastfeeding mothers continued to take the same capsules for six months; bottle-fed infants were given the probiotics or placebo directly. Over the next two years, the babies received thorough physical examinations and the mothers were questioned about any symptoms.

Forty-six per cent of the babies in the placebo group developed eczema. This number may seem high, but remember that these infants were at risk for the condition because of their family history. However, only 23 per cent of those who received probiotics showed any signs of the disease – a striking difference. The findings were published in 2001 in the prestigious British medical journal *The Lancet*, with an accompanying editorial by Dr Simon Murch of the Centre for Paediatric Gastroenterology, Royal Free and University College School of Medicine, London. Dr Murch noted, 'These figures are remarkable and, if confirmed in other studies and applicable to other allergic diseases, probiotics would represent an important therapeutic advance.'

Two other studies by the same team of Finnish investigators demonstrated that probiotics could help infants who already had atopic dermatitis. One of these investigations treated babies by adding the probiotic *Lactobacillus rhamnosus* GG to their formula. After just one month, atopic dermatitis in those babies was significantly diminished compared with that of untreated infants. The second study tested another probiotic, *Bifidobacterium lactis* Bb-12, as well as *L. rhamnosus* GG, with similar therapeutic results. Babies in the second study were followed up at the age of 4. Those who had been treated with probiotics had half the rate of atopic dermatitis compared with the group that had not received probiotics during infancy. Additional studies are under way to confirm these results and to explore other probiotic regimens that could prevent or treat atopic dermatitis.

FOOD ALLERGIES

According to the National Institute of Allergy and Infectious Diseases, one out of three people report that they have a food allergy – but most of them are wrong. Technically speaking, a food allergy is an immune response against some molecule in food. Usually, what people casually call a food allergy is really a food intolerance – namely, an adverse reaction to a particular food. (See the box on the next page.)

It's easy to understand why the two would be confused. Food intolerances produce symptoms similar to those of food allergies. However, the difference is that these reactions don't directly involve the immune system. True allergic reactions to foods are rare: only about 6 to 8 per cent of children have them and the problem is even less common in adults.

Symptoms and the Usual Treatment

With food allergies, as with other allergies, the immune system reacts to a harmless substance as if it were a dangerous microbe, releasing histamine. In theory, any food can trigger an allergic response. In practice, however, about 90 per cent of food allergies are accounted for by these eight categories: milk, eggs, wheat, soya, peanuts, nuts that grow on trees (almonds, cashews, etc.), fish and shellfish.

The standard treatment for a food allergy – and the only currently available preventive measure – is simple: don't eat the offending food. If the cause isn't obvious, keeping a food diary (be sure to include beverages) and recording any symptoms can help you to track down the culprit.

Just because treatment is simple doesn't mean it's easy. Giving up foods you enjoy is hard enough. But far more difficult is

➤ FOOD INTOLERANCES ➤

Allergic reactions aren't the only reason that a particular food might disagree with us. Food intolerances and sensitivities can stimulate a variety of unpleasant effects in the body – including some that are similar to those of food allergies. A few examples are:

• **Lactose intolerance:** If you're deficient in the enzyme that digests lactose, the sugar in milk, you may experience wind, diarrhoea or nausea when you consume dairy products. Good news: probiotics help break down lactose, which means that some people who can't tolerate other dairy foods have no problem with yoghurt or aged cheese. (See Chapter 10, page 226, for more on lactose intolerance.)

• **Sensitivity to caffeine:** Coffee, tea, chocolate and many fizzy beverages contain caffeine. For some, it's a pleasant pick-me-up. But others may experience adverse effects, including rapid heartbeat and tremors, especially if they overdo it.

• **Reactions to monosodium glutamate (MSG):** So-called Chinese restaurant syndrome – hot flushes, sweating, headache and a feeling of pressure in the face – is caused by an adverse reaction to MSG, a flavour enhancer that's used not only in Chinese restaurants but also in many processed foods.

avoiding hidden sources of allergens. For instance, who would think that tins of tuna could present a problem for someone with a milk allergy? But some tinned tuna contains casein, a milk protein.

Seemingly plain chocolate might pick up trace amounts of peanuts from other sweets processed on the same equipment, thereby endangering a person who is highly sensitive to peanuts.

If a triggering food is consumed, the immediate symptoms usually involve itchy skin or swelling in the lips, mouth, tongue and throat. Other reactions can occur later, such as a runny nose, shortness of breath, dizziness or skin reactions like hives, hot flushes or a rash. Vomiting or diarrhoea is also possible. Relatively mild reactions like these are treated with antihistamines and measures to address specific symptoms, such as a skin cream for itching.

Much less common – and far more dangerous – is a severe allergic reaction called anaphylaxis. Within minutes of consuming a triggering food, the mast cells of a highly allergic person can release exceptionally large amounts of histamine, which makes blood vessels dilate. Blood pressure drops and at the same time tissues become swollen throughout the body. Significant inflammation in the nose and throat can actually cut off the air supply. Anaphylaxis is life-threatening. Athough firm statistics are hard to come by, one in 100 children in the UK is believed to suffer severe allergic reactions to peanuts, tree nuts, or both.

Anaphylaxis is treated with epinephrine (adrenaline), a hormone that rapidly reverses the effects of histamine: it constricts dilated blood vessels, stimulates the heart to build blood pressure, counters swelling and relaxes muscles in the airways to help open constricted passageways. Because an anaphylactic reaction may develop too quickly for the victim to seek medical assistance, those at risk are urged to carry a device (such as an EpiPen) that allows them to quickly inject themselves with epinephrine. However, the emergency doesn't end with the injection. Though epinephrine is a lifesaving drug, its side effects can be severe, including heart palpitations, difficulty breathing and vomiting. All this underscores the importance of preventing allergic reactions.

Emerging Evidence for Probiotics

Research in animals has shown that probiotic supplements can significantly decrease allergic responses to food. Scientists can create allergies in mice and other laboratory animals by feeding them a particular food along with chemicals that irritate the intestinal lining. Because the immune system detects both the food and nearby damage, it treats the food as if it were a dangerous microbe and generates an immune response. Laboratory research supports the idea that probiotics – by controlling inflammation – could prevent development of allergies.

In one study, investigators at Seoul National University in South Korea used this technique to make two groups of mice allergic to chicken egg white, a common human food allergen. At the same time, mice in one group were given probiotic supplements containing *Bifidobacterium bifidum* BGN4 and *Lactobacillus casei* 911; the other mice received no probiotics. Five weeks later, they fed chicken egg white to all the mice. The question was: could probiotic bacteria somehow thwart the researchers' efforts to create an egg white allergy? The answer: yes. Those treated with probiotics had significantly decreased allergic reactivity – as measured by histamine release from mast cells and other allergic responses – compared with the untreated mice. The findings were published in 2005 in *FEMS Immunology and Medical Microbiology*, a journal of the Federation of European Microbiological Societies.

Findings like these have encouraged researchers to conduct human trials that explore the potential of probiotics in preventing food allergies. For example, two separate studies in infants have shown promise for reducing milk allergies by giving babies supplements of *Lactobacillus rhamnosus* GG.

In one of these investigations, Finnish scientists studied 27 infants who suffered from atopic eczema that was exacerbated by an allergy to cow's milk. For one month, cow's milk was removed from their diets. At the same time, 13 of the babies were given *Lacto-bacillus* GG in a formula known to be tolerated by infants allergic to cow's milk; the other 14 participants received the same formula, but without probiotic bacteria. A standard scoring system was used to assess the severity of the babies' eczema before and after this experiment. After one month, the infants receiving the probiotic showed significant improvement of their eczema compared with those who received ordinary formula. The findings were published in 1997 in the *Journal of Allergy and Clinical Immunology.* A subsequent larger study of 230 infants with suspected allergy to milk, published in 2005 in *Allergy*, also showed that consumption of *Lactobacillus rhamnosus* GG could significantly reduce atopic eczema.

We don't yet know nearly as much about food allergies as we do about allergies that affect the respiratory system. But initial research is so promising that answers should be coming soon. Meanwhile, I think probiotics are worth a try, both to treat allergies and to prevent them. Your best bet is to consume a variety of probiotic microbes; if you don't get the desired results, try a different combination.

SINUSITIS

The sinuses (or, to use the correct term, the paranasal sinuses) are hollow spaces in the skull that are joined to the nose. Like the nose, the sinuses are lined with mucosal surfaces. They're used both to humidify the air we breathe and to trap airborne particles in mucus.

In sinusitis, the lining of the sinuses becomes inflamed. A typical case starts with a viral infection, such as a cold. The immune system reacts with inflammation and increased mucus production. Ordinarily, excess mucus would drain out through the nose, but swollen tissues may prevent that. If fluid builds up in the sinuses, bacteria that are normally present in low numbers may multiply and cause an infection.

People with sinusitis find it difficult – sometimes impossible – to breathe through the nose. What's more, the pressure of fluid accumulation in the sinuses often causes painful headaches. These debilitating problems may be accompanied by fever, fatigue and overall weakness.

Sinusitis can be acute, meaning that it lasts for only a week or so. Some people – such as those with allergic rhinitis – may experience frequent bouts of acute sinusitis. But sinusitis may become chronic, in which case congestion and inflammation of the mucosal surfaces never goes away. Uncontrolled inflammation can destroy tissue or lead to polyps – benign grape-shaped growths – on the mucosa. If the polyps are large enough, they further obstruct the flow of air. Acute sinusitis affects three in 1,000 people in the United Kingdom. Chronic sinusitis affects one in 1,000 people. Sinusitis is more common in winter than in summer.

Conventional Treatments

The treatments that get patients past an attack of acute sinusitis – decongestants and antibiotics (if there's a bacterial infection) – aren't always effective for chronic sinusitis. Moreover, these drugs can have troubling side effects if used constantly.

Sometimes steroid nasal sprays are prescribed when sinusitis becomes chronic, but these also have troublesome side effects. Surgery – performed to remove large polyps or to open passage-ways – is considered a last resort.

A SINUS SPECIALIST SPEAKS ABOUT PROBIOTICS

Otolaryngologist Jeffrey E. Terrell, MD, directs the Michigan Sinus Center at the University of Michigan. Here's what he recommends to patients taking antibiotics:

I treat patients with chronic and acute sinusitis, who go on oral antibiotics for three to four weeks. Antibiotics kill the normal intestinal flora. As a result, a fair number of my patients get antibiotic-associated simple diarrhoea or C. difficile diarrhoea. Either is a problem, but C. difficile can cause substantial complications of the large intestine, so it's nice to be able to avoid it. I tell patients to take a yoghurt with active cultures or to take acidophilus supplements. When they do that, I don't hear about as many problems.

The Possible Role of Probiotics

Probiotics can head off antibiotic side effects during sinusitis treatment. Could they be used to prevent or cure the disease? Recently, our laboratory made a startling observation in mice that suggests a link between chronic sinusitis and an unbalanced gut microflora. If these are indeed connected, then restoring the microflora with probiotics might prove therapeutic.

We worked with two groups of mice. One group received a treatment designed to disrupt their normal microflora. First we gave these mice a broad-spectrum antibiotic to destroy most of the bacteria in their gut, including the probiotics. Before we stopped the antibiotic, we allowed the yeast *Candida albicans*, which is normally kept in check by competition with other microbes, to flourish in their intestines. The other group of mice was left untreated. Both groups were fed the same food and they lived in the same environment.

In our lab, mice are housed in clean cages whose floor is lined with ground corncobs. The untreated mice remained healthy in this environment. However, within a week after the treatment that altered their gut microflora, the other mice spontaneously developed chronic sinusitis, probably as an allergic reaction to some substance inhaled from the corncobs. This experiment showed that decimating the population of probiotic bacteria, and disrupting the balance of the microflora in the body, can lead to chronic sinusitis.

One of the key functions of probiotics is to support immuno-logic tolerance. Without adequate probiotics, the antibiotic-treated mice lost their normal immunologic tolerance to something inhaled from their environment. We plan research to test the hypothesis that adding probiotics to the diet – thereby restoring immune tolerance – will decrease their sinusitis. After all, sinusitis is an inflammatory disease of the mucosa, just like inflammatory bowel disease (IBD). We know that the inflammation of IBD is turned off when probiotics are used to stimulate the action of regulatory T cells. So we strongly suspect that the same mechanism will work for chronic sinusitis, too.

I know from personal experience how miserable and frustrating it is to suffer from allergies. A person with allergies can't tolerate aspects of everyday life that most people take for granted. Almost anything – a friendly dog, a bouquet of flowers, a packet of peanuts – can set off uncomfortable, embarrassing and even dangerous reactions. Ordinary chores, like sweeping or doing the laundry, may produce debilitating symptoms. Sometimes the only safe treatment is to curtail normal activities. Allergies can make you feel like a prisoner.

Research is just beginning to show that probiotics can prevent and treat a wide variety of allergies. While scientists investigate further, you don't have to wait for their results. As I described in Chapter 1, I've used a combination of healthy dietary modifications, plus daily probiotic supplements, to all but cure the allergic rhinitis from which I've suffered since childhood. In Part 3, I'll explain how you can do the same.

CHAPTER EIGHT

Urogenital Diseases

E merging research suggests that probiotics can help to prevent and treat three common conditions that affect the urinary and genital organs: vaginitis, urinary tract infections and kidney stones. And what a relief that would be! These difficulties affect millions of people, especially women. Though rarely life-threatening, they're frequently annoying, painful and debilitating. Prevention is particularly important with all three, because the problems tend to recur. And the most common medical treatments – systemic antibiotics or antifungal medications – create problems of their own by destroying friendly microbes along with harmful ones. Consuming probiotics during treatment can offset these negative side effects as well.

VAGINITIS

Vaginitis refers to an inflammation of the vaginal lining. The condition can be asymptomatic, but usually it produces such problems as an abnormal vaginal discharge, unpleasant odour and irritation, itching, burning or pain. The problem is a very common one among women in the United Kingdom, accounting for thousands of doctor visits each year.

The two most common causes of vaginitis are infections from bacteria and from the yeast *Candida albicans*. Vaginitis also can be caused by a parasite called *Trichomonas*, by viruses or by irritants such as contraceptive creams, bubble bath or detergents used to wash underwear. Since these situations require different treatments, getting an accurate diagnosis is the first step in addressing vaginitis. Women sometimes suffer longer than necessary because they take a medication that has worked with similar symptoms in the past, but that isn't appropriate for the particular type of vaginitis they have now.

Bacterial Vaginosis

Certain microbes normally live in the vagina, including probiotic *Lactobacilli* bacteria. As with the digestive tract, the vaginal microflora is normally in a healthy balance that keeps disease-causing microbes in check. But this balance can be disrupted by a variety of factors. A woman may be exposed to sexually transmitted bacteria, such as *Chlamydia*, that cause vaginal inflammation. Sometimes the microflora is adversely affected by antibiotics or other medications, particularly ones given vaginally – including contraceptive cream. Hormonal changes can also affect the vaginal microflora. That's why women are vulnerable to infections during pregnancy or the menopause.

Whatever the cause of the disruption, harmful bacteria, which usually live in low numbers in the vagina, seize the opportunity to proliferate. The most common symptoms of bacterial vaginosis are itching, irritation and a discharge with a fishy odour. Diagnosis is confirmed by microscopic examination of vaginal discharge. Typically, the condition is treated with antibiotics, which the patient takes orally or in the form of a vaginal cream or gel.

Yeast Infections

The same disruptions in the vaginal microflora that open the door to bacterial vaginosis also can permit the overgrowth of yeast. The yeast most likely to cause a vaginal infection is *Candida albicans*. Experts estimate that three out of four women will experience at least one *C. albicans* infection during their lifetime. The problem is a common side effect of antibiotic treatment.

Typical symptoms include a white discharge, burning during urination, itching and soreness. The discharge is examined under a microscope to confirm the cause. Yeast infections are treated with antifungal medications, such as miconazole or clotrimazole, usually given as a vaginal cream or suppository. Another option, which is not available to pregnant women because of possible risks to the baby, is an oral antifungal drug.

The Evidence for Probiotics

Since many vaginal infections result from an unbalanced microflora, there's been considerable interest in using probiotics to prevent these problems. Research first focused on identifying probiotic strains that can survive and grow in the vagina. Microbes that normally live in the digestive tract don't necessarily flourish if transplanted to another part of the body. For example, *Lactobacillus rhamnosus* GG – a probiotic used to treat gastrointestinal disorders – doesn't thrive in the vagina, even when directly introduced via suppositories. However, other *Lactobacillus* strains, including *L. rhamnosus* GR-1 and *L. fermentum* RC 14, will colonise the vagina after being taken orally.

The next question was whether these probiotics could counter the bacteria and yeast that cause vaginitis. Though the evidence is not yet conclusive, some clinical trials have shown that certain lactic acid bacteria – including *L. acidophilus*, *L. rhamnosus* GR-1 and *L. fermentum* RC-14 – can prevent vaginitis. These studies have administered probiotics either orally or via vaginal suppositories. Also under investigation is the possibility of using panty liners impregnated with probiotics.

Probiotics work by competing with the bacteria and yeast that cause vaginal infections, keeping their populations low. The option of using probiotics is especially attractive for women who have experienced adverse reactions to medications normally prescribed to prevent these infections, or who have other contraindications for using them.

URINARY TRACT INFECTIONS

The urinary tract starts with the kidneys. These twin organs maintain a healthy balance of water in the body. As they remove excess water from the bloodstream, they filter out waste products produced by our cells; these wastes are collected in the urine. The kidneys create urine continuously. It flows to the bladder for storage via tubes called ureters. When the bladder becomes full, we empty it, urinating via the urethra.

We don't think of urine as sterile, but it is if we're healthy. Nevertheless, the urinary tract – from kidneys to urethra – is vulnerable to infection by microbes from the digestive tract. The most frequent culprit is *E. coli*, but it's not the only one.

Urinary tract infections (UTIs) are a common problem, accounting for thousands of doctor visits each year in the United

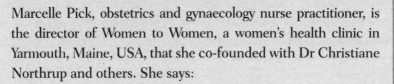
A NURSE PRACTITIONER SPEAKS ABOUT CHRONIC YEAST INFECTIONS

Marcelle Pick, obstetrics and gynaecology nurse practitioner, is the director of Women to Women, a women's health clinic in Yarmouth, Maine, USA, that she co-founded with Dr Christiane Northrup and others. She says:

Women from all over the country with chronic yeast infections come to see me. A simple stool test can be done to determine if a patient has yeast overgrowth. I know that there is controversy about this – some practitioners clearly disagree with the notion of systemic yeast. I can tell you from treating thousands of women who have suffered for years with this issue – it is real, and yes, it can be treated effectively.

At Women to Women, we tackle yeast vaginitis with a three-step approach. First we recommend a sugar-free diet. Then we use an antimicrobial to decrease the yeast. We also put them on a probiotic three times a day. This provides a natural remedy. Our patients see results. Their symptoms go away and they feel great!

Kingdom. Approximately 20 per cent of women develop a UTI at some time in their lives; once they do, the problem is likely to recur. Men are much less vulnerable to these infections, though this changes late in life. Experts speculate that anatomy accounts for these differences. Women, whose urethra is closer to the anal opening, are more likely to become infected. But since urine helps flush bacteria from the urinary tract, anything that obstructs the flow can lead to a UTI. That includes an enlarged prostate gland, which is a common condition in older men.

If the problem is confined to the lower part of the urinary tract, the symptoms may be relatively mild – unusually frequent urination, sometimes with pain or burning. But if the infection reaches the kidneys, it can cause severe pain, nausea, fever and significant malaise. Infected kidneys can be damaged permanently unless the condition is addressed.

Conventional Medical Approaches

Treatment usually begins with a urine test to identify the bacterium responsible for an infection, and then an appropriate antibiotic is prescribed. Painkillers may be needed as well. When the UTI is not severe, symptoms often disappear a day or two after treatment starts. However, the bacteria may linger longer. Follow-up urine tests are recommended to make sure the infection is gone before medication is discontinued.

Recurrent UTIs are a common problem. Some women have three or more recurrences per year. Whatever caused one infection can produce others. Risk factors include diabetes, medication that suppresses the immune system and use of a diaphragm for contraception. Sometimes the problem is caused by anatomical abnormalities. Anyone who experiences frequent UTIs should see a urinary disorder or kidney specialist for evaluation.

Preventing recurrences is especially important because there's a danger of kidney involvement. Recommended lifestyle adjustments include drinking plenty of fluids and emptying the bladder as soon as it feels full. The most commonly prescribed preventive measure is low doses of antibiotics, taken daily for six months or even longer. Ironically, this increases the risk of a vaginal yeast infection and possibly of a kidney stone, as I'll explain below. Fortunately, these risks can be countered by probiotics. (See pages 242–243 in Chapter 11 for information on consuming probiotics to restore the microflora when you're taking antibiotics.)

➤➤ THE CRANBERRY JUICE OPTION ➤➤

You've probably heard that cranberry juice can prevent urinary tract infections. It's true. When the connection was first discovered, scientists assumed that the acidity of the juice was responsible. We now realise that credit should also go to proanthocyanidin, a prebiotic compound found in cranberries. It supports probiotics – and helps ward off UTIs – by preventing *E. coli* from attaching to the cells that line the urethra and bladder. When *E. coli* can't cling to the walls of the urinary tract, they're swept away by the normal flow of urine.

How much cranberry juice must you drink to keep UTIs at bay? Unfortunately, no one knows for sure. In a 2004 review article for *American Family Physician*, author Darren M Lynch, MD, of the Northampton Wellness Associates in Northampton, Massachusetts, USA, recommended one tablet of concentrated cranberry extract (300 to 400 milligrams) twice daily, or 240 ml of pure unsweetened cranberry juice three times daily. This advice was based on the most recent successful randomised controlled trial.

Dr Lynch noted that although studies that follow subjects for up to twelve months have found that regular cranberry consumption is safe, care should be taken in recommending long-term use in people who have a history of kidney stones. That's because cranberries contain oxalate, a chemical that can create kidney stones when it combines with calcium. However, certain probiotics may help to reduce this risk, as explained later in this chapter.

The Probiotic Connection

Medical researchers have known for decades that there's a connection between recurrent UTIs in women and the number of probiotic *Lactobacillus* bacteria in their vaginas. Those with low *Lactobacilli* counts have an increased risk of these infections, while those whose *Lactobacilli* counts are high are more likely to have a healthy urinary tract.

Does this mean that consuming probiotics can prevent urinary tract infections? Though definitive clinical trials have yet to be reported, preliminary studies suggest that it's possible. For example, Finnish investigators compared 139 women who were suffering from a UTI with 185 age-matched women who had been free of UTIs for the previous five years. All the women were questioned in detail about their diets. Those with a healthy urinary tract were significantly more likely to eat or drink fermented milk products at least three times a week – and they also reported a higher consumption of berry juices, which help to support probiotics.

KIDNEY STONES

The pain from a kidney stone can be worse than that of childbirth, report women who have experienced both. Urine contains minerals and other substances that can form tiny crystals inside the kidneys. These crystals may become larger or combine, forming a hard stone. If it's small enough, a crystal or stone is simply carried out of the kidneys by the normal flow of urine. But larger stones may irritate the kidneys and urinary tract – or even create blockages. Apart from pain, a stone can cause an infection or damage to the kidney.

According to statistics from the National Institutes of Health, more than 5 per cent of Americans have had kidney stones. They prompt about 2.7 million consultations with healthcare providers annually and more than 600,000 visits to A&E. Men are more likely to develop the problem than women are – and anyone who has had kidney stones in the past is vulnerable to a recurrence. Preliminary research suggests that certain probiotics may help to prevent the most common type of kidney stone.

Diagnosis and Treatment

A kidney stone that produces severe pain is readily diagnosed by an X-ray, CT scan, or ultrasound. However, some kidney stones are asymptomatic. They are found after routine tests reveal blood in the urine, or they are discovered when the imaging tests mentioned above are performed to investigate other problems.

If the stone is small enough to pass through the urinary tract without causing damage – which is often the case – the only treatment suggested may be drinking extra water to speed the process along. Otherwise, one of the following procedures can be used to destroy or remove the stone:

- **Shock waves** (called extracorporeal shockwave lithotripsy): A machine beams shock waves at the stone, breaking it into pieces small enough to exit through the urinary tract. This is the most common approach to stones that are too large to pass on their own.
- **Tunnel surgery** (called percutaneous nephrolithotomy): A tunnel-like device is inserted into the kidney through the back. Then the surgeon sends a special viewing and operating instrument through the tunnel to find and remove the stone. This procedure is used for larger kidney stones.
- **Ureteroscopic stone removal**: Instead of operating through the back, the surgeon threads a viewing instrument through the urethra and into the urinary tract. This device, called a uretero-scope, permits the surgeon to remove or shatter the stone.

What Causes Kidney Stones?

The most common type of kidney stone is made from calcium oxalate, a compound made up of two substances – calcium and oxalate – that all of us consume in our diet. Oxalate is found in many common plant foods; it's also produced during the normal metabolism of dietary sugars and amino acids. However, if the oxalate level in the body becomes too high, it can accumulate and possibly combine with calcium to form kidney stones. Less commonly, kidney stones are made from other chemical combinations. They also may develop as a result of urinary tract infections, kidney disease or certain unusual metabolic disorders.

When kidney stones have a known medical cause, addressing the problem can prevent recurrences. Medication – including low-dose antibiotics for certain types of kidney stones – may be used to alter the chemical composition of a person's urine. Otherwise, the conventional approach to prevention is to make lifestyle changes. Everyone at risk for a recurrence is advised to drink plenty of liquids. Those who form calcium oxalate stones may be told to cut back on foods containing oxalate, including spinach, beets, strawberries, tea and nuts.

Preventing Kidney Stones with Probiotics

People with high levels of oxalate in their urine are at risk for kidney stones. The presence of this chemical suggests that the body isn't metabolising it properly. Most substances that we consume are broken down by digestive enzymes that our body makes. But oxalate is different. The enzyme needed to digest it isn't made by us, but by bacteria in our microflora, most notably the probiotic *Oxalobacter formigenes*, which normally lives in our gut. If the oxalate isn't broken down in the intestinal tract, the kidneys must try to filter it out – and if oxalate levels become high, stones may form in the kidneys.

Studies find that people who form oxalate-containing kidney stones are far more likely to have very low levels of *O. formigenes* than are healthy individuals. Long-term use of antibiotics – prescribed for many reasons, including prevention of recurrent urinary tract infections – is associated with an absence of *O. formigenes*. Scientists have speculated that prolonged antibiotic exposure might increase the chances of getting a kidney stone.

Preliminary investigations in both animals and humans indicate that administering *O. formigenes* reduces the level of oxalate in the blood and urine – an effect that suggests it could help to prevent kidney stones. This particular probiotic isn't yet available commercially. But the same enzyme that *O. formigenes* makes to break down oxalate in the intestines is produced by other probiotic bacteria – including *Bifidobacterium lactis*, *B. infantis* and *Lactobacillus acidophilus* – that are found in some yoghurts and supplements.

Research is ongoing to determine which probiotics might help to prevent and treat urogenital disease, and how best to use them. In the meantime, if you've been plagued by these conditions, consider adding probiotics to other suggested measures – such as drinking more water and avoiding irritants – to reduce the chances of recurrence.

CHAPTER NINE

A Glimpse of the Future

Often, when I read about complex and baffling medical conditions whose causes are not fully understood, I wonder if there might be a microflora connection – even if no one has yet proposed the idea. My index of suspicion shoots up when the condition involves gastrointestinal symptoms or when inflammation seems to play a role. I'm also intrigued if the people who have these conditions tend to suffer from other problems, such as irritable bowel syndrome, where there's already evidence that the microflora are involved.

When I explore the scientific and medical literature, I frequently find relevant animal studies that show the promise of probiotics. Sometimes I turn up investigations in humans that weren't designed to study probiotics but that offer intriguing hints suggesting they might have therapeutic benefits. In this chapter, I invite you to share my excitement about these possibilities.

AUTOIMMUNE DISEASES

In an autoimmune disease, the body wages war against itself. The immune system strikes out against our own cells, destroying tissue and causing loss of function. It could happen to any organ or tissue in the body. Inflammatory bowel disease was described in Chapter 6; other autoimmune diseases are listed in the table on the following page. But those are just some familiar examples. More than eighty different autoimmune conditions have been identified. Some are so rare that few doctors have ever encountered them. Collectively, though, they're anything but rare: an estimated 5 to 8 per cent of Americans — 14 to 22 million people – suffer from an autoimmune disease, according to the Autoimmune Diseases Coordinating Committee of the National Institutes of Health.

Autoimmunity isn't like other diseases, which have a clear pattern of symptoms. It takes a bewildering variety of forms, depending upon the particular tissue that's attacked. Who would think that the same basic malfunction could cause the crippling effects of multiple sclerosis, the skin lesions of psoriasis and the bulging eyes that are the hallmark of Graves' disease?

If you check the areas of expertise recognised by the American Board of Medical Specialties, you won't find autoimmunity on the list. Typically, patients with these conditions seek treatment from their primary care provider or from whatever medical specialist seems appropriate for their chief symptom – a gastroenterologist for IBD, a dermatologist for scleroderma. But autoimmunity also involves chronic inflammation and associated systemic reactions. What's more, a person with one autoimmune disease is susceptible

AUTOIMMUNE DISEASES

These are just some of the eighty-plus autoimmune diseases identified so far.

NAME	TARGET	COMMON SYMPTOMS
Inflammatory bowel disease	Intestines	Diarrhoea, abdominal pain, fatigu
Rheumatoid arthritis	Lining of joints throughout the body	Joint pain and stiffness
Type 1 diabetes	Insulin-producing cells in the pancreas	Dangerously high blood sugar
Multiple sclerosis	Tissue that surrounds nerves	Numbness, weakness, vision problems
Lupus	Skin, joints, blood vessels, kidneys and other organs	Joint pain, fatigue, skin rashes
Psoriasis	Skin tissue	Skin lesions
Scleroderma	Skin and connective tissue	Thickening and hardening of the skin
Sjögren's syndrome	Moisture-producing glands in the body, especially the eyes	Dry eyes
Graves' disease	Thyroid gland	Overproduction of thyroid hormon
Hashimoto's disease	Thyroid gland	Underproduction of thyroid horma
Glomerulonephritis	Kidneys	Kidney failure
Guillain-Barré syndrome	Peripheral nervous system	Weakness, numbness, paralysis

to another. Symptoms can confuse even caring, experienced phy
cians. According to a survey by the American Autoimmune Rela
Diseases Association, most people who eventually were found to h
an autoimmune disease received at least one incorrect diagno
first. Many were told that their symptoms simply reflected stre

Shockingly, nearly half of those surveyed had been labelled hypo-chondriacs before their disease was properly identified.

The common features of autoimmune disorders haven't always been appreciated. But that's changing. New research on inflamma-tion has inspired new thinking about these diseases. Furthermore, some medical experts are beginning to suspect that other condi-tions whose origins are not yet clear – including autism and chronic fatigue syndrome – might involve inflammation and autoimmunity.

So far, IBD is the only autoimmune condition for which human studies of probiotics have been done. But it's only a matter of time. Research with animals has begun and the findings so far are highly promising.

The Common Features of Autoimmune Diseases

Though each autoimmune disease has unique symptoms, all of them have one thing in common: chronic inflammation. For reasons that are not yet understood, the regulatory T cells – whose activity I described in Chapter 4 – fail to perform their normal job of turning off inflammation. Consequently, helper T cells enter the affected tissue and direct an inflammatory response that continues even after it has become destructive.

People with an autoimmune disease must deal with much more than the consequences of specific tissue damage. Inflammation also causes multiple systemic reactions – fever, exhaustion, depression and muscle or joint pain. Life becomes unpredictable. Episodes of acute symptoms are followed by periods of remission, only to return without warning. Relapses might occur in response to an infection, stress or a dietary change. Inflammation anywhere in the body – even if unrelated to the autoimmune disease – can trigger a flare-up.

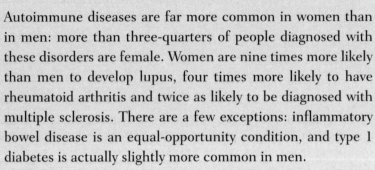

AUTOIMMUNITY: A WOMEN'S HEALTH ISSUE

Autoimmune diseases are far more common in women than in men: more than three-quarters of people diagnosed with these disorders are female. Women are nine times more likely than men to develop lupus, four times more likely to have rheumatoid arthritis and twice as likely to be diagnosed with multiple sclerosis. There are a few exceptions: inflammatory bowel disease is an equal-opportunity condition, and type 1 diabetes is actually slightly more common in men.

Should we blame oestrogen and other sex hormones? Probably. Most women are diagnosed during their reproductive years. However, some autoimmune conditions improve during pregnancy, whereas others become worse.

We know that oestrogen can affect the immune system directly. There's also evidence that oestrogen has indirect effects via its impact on the microflora. For example, yeast infections are far more prevalent during pregnancy than at other times in a woman's life. That's because the yeasts that cause infections are better able to adhere to the intestinal tract and to other cells in the presence of oestrogen.

Researchers are still exploring this chain of influences – from oestrogen affecting yeast and other microbes, to imbalances in the microflora, to autoimmune conditions – and the results aren't in yet. Nonetheless, it makes sense for women with a personal or family history of these diseases to consider consuming probiotics as a safe and effective way to promote a healthy immune system.

The Microflora Hypothesis and Autoimmunity

I strongly suspect that imbalances in the gut microflora make us more vulnerable to autoimmunity, just as they do with allergies. I'm intrigued by the fact that the rise of asthma (an allergic disease) is correlated with the increase in type 1 diabetes (an autoimmune condition) in industrialised countries during the last four decades. The explanation could be found in the microflora hypothesis, which I described in Chapter 7: exposure to probiotic microbes is essential to the healthy development of the immune system.

In autoimmune diseases, as in allergies, the immune system targets a harmless substance, producing chronic inflammation and associated symptoms. Regulatory T cells fail to turn off unnecessary immune responses – a problem that we've already shown to be linked to insufficient probiotic microbes in the gut microflora.

We know that autoimmune conditions tend to run in families. However, the disease itself is usually not what's inherited. Rather, there are problems in one or more of the many genes that regulate immune responses. Similarly, we know that some autoimmune diseases appear to be triggered by infections. As I explained in Chapter 4, the immune system may target one of the body's own cells, simply because it looks similar to the infectious microbe – the phenomenon called molecular mimicry. Even after the original infection disappears, the autoimmune reaction can persist.

The Long-Term Treatment Dilemma

People with autoimmune diseases face a troubling dilemma. Once established, most of these diseases are chronic, lifelong conditions. But the most effective treatments often come with dangerous or debilitating side effects.

These conditions are treated in different ways. One treatment avenue targets the underlying inflammation and problematic immune responses. Mild inflammation can be addressed with aspirin and other non-steroidal anti-inflammatory drugs. More significant inflammation requires steroids or immunosuppressive drugs. But these powerful medications come with side effects. And any drug that suppresses the immune system raises the risk of infection.

In Hashimoto's disease (which interferes with the production of thyroid hormone) and type 1 diabetes (which destroys insulin-producing cells in the pancreas), treatment involves daily use of artificial replacement hormones. Some treatments for other autoimmune diseases simply focus on relieving symptoms. For example, physical therapy and exercise address the stiffness of conditions like rheumatoid arthritis, multiple sclerosis and lupus.

Since probiotics are safe to take on a long-term basis, they're an especially attractive option for use with other therapies in treating autoimmune conditions. Probiotics are already recommended as a supplement to antibiotic treatment for inflammatory bowel disease. And there's much more to come. Researchers have taken crucial first steps towards truly innovative therapies that could actually prevent and cure these conditions: animal studies.

From the Laboratory to the Chemist

In the late 1980s, when I was a graduate student at the University of Texas Southwestern Medical School, our immunology programme was at the forefront of efforts to understand the underlying causes of autoimmune diseases. A remarkable new technology had just been developed, which enabled scientists to move a gene from one organism to another – even if the two organisms were of different species. Faculty members at the University of Texas Southwestern Medical School decided to use this transgenic technology to create rats with a human gene – HLA-B27 – that's strongly associated with vulnerability to colitis, rheumatoid arthritis and other autoimmune diseases.

They obtained fertilised eggs from pregnant rats by the same methods used for harvesting human fertilised eggs for assisted reproduction. They isolated HLA-B27 genes from a sample of human white blood cells. Using a tiny needle, they injected an HLA-B27 gene into each rat egg; then they returned the eggs to their mothers' wombs. Inside the eggs, the human gene joined the rat DNA. When the pups were born, they looked like any other newborn rats and were rat-like in every respect – except (as was verified by examining their DNA) for having one human gene.

The HLA-B27 rats were among the first transgenic laboratory animals to be created, so everyone at our school was interested in them. But what really generated excitement was not merely that the rats possessed a human gene, but that the gene worked the same way in the rats as it does in people who have it. I still remember attending a seminar at which the first studies with these rats were presented. The researchers showed slides of biopsies taken from the joints and intestinal tracts of normal rats and HLA-B27 rats. What a difference! The tissues of the HLA-B27 rats were red and inflamed. Their immune systems had spontaneously attacked their own bodies, and these rats had developed rheumatoid arthritis and ulcerative colitis.

Why was this so exciting? Finally, we could observe the actual disease process in an animal, not a Petri dish, and show that the suspected gene was really involved. Animal models, such as the HLA-B27 rats, also greatly accelerate the progress of medical research. Many of these diseases don't strike until adulthood – a long time to wait in humans, but a matter of months in rats and mice.

Nearly two decades after graduate school, I'm still intrigued by the potential of specially bred mice. My laboratory is working on creating healthy mice with a made-to-order microflora that will open new avenues for research. Instead of hosting hundreds of different microbes in their intestines, these mice will have just fifteen to twenty. By reducing the number of microbes, we'll be able to take a closer look at their interactions and at the effects they have on the immune system and the body.

The Probiotics Connection

By now, many scientists have worked with the HLA-B27 rats, attempting to find improved therapies for the autoimmune conditions to which they're so vulnerable. In one investigation, scientists from the University of North Carolina followed an antibiotic treatment protocol that's known to be effective in humans with inflammatory bowel disease. While this can bring HLA-B27 rats (and humans) into remission, symptoms usually recur when the drugs are discontinued. After the rats were taken off antibiotics, some were given a probiotic (*Lactobacillus rhamnosus* GG). Those that didn't receive the probiotic had the expected relapse. But the HLA-B27 rats that consumed the probiotic remained in remission. This was a significant finding: even animals that are genetically programmed to develop a chronic autoimmune disease can be spared by taking probiotics.

Another experiment involving probiotics used specially bred mice – called NOD (non-obese diabetic) mice – that are genetically destined to have a very high risk of developing type 1 diabetes. These mice don't properly generate the regulatory responses that turn off unnecessary immune reactions. By the time they reach the age of six months, over 75 per cent of the females and 20 per cent of the males have developed type 1 diabetes.

In an Italian study, however, researchers were able to prevent this condition in NOD mice by giving them the supplement called VSL#3, which contains a blend of probiotic *Bifidobacterium*, *Lactobacillus* and *Streptococcus* strains. The investigators also demonstrated that the mice given VSL#3 developed regulatory responses, while the controls did not. This explains how the probiotics protected so many of these vulnerable mice from type 1 diabetes.

In 2000, congressional legislation in the USA established a permanent Autoimmune Disease Coordinating Committee within the National Institutes of Health (NIH). Two years later, the committee issued an ambitious research plan to address auto-immune diseases in the United States. Reading the plan, I was particularly struck by this observation:

> *Researchers are only beginning to grasp the complexity of regulatory cell control of autoimmune responses. By under-standing how to induce regulatory responses, it may be possible to prevent autoimmune diseases as well as to treat them.*

We know that probiotics are strong stimulators of regulatory immune responses. That's why they hold so much promise for preventing and treating autoimmunity. The animal studies I've described – which have successfully used probiotics to prevent autoimmune conditions, even in the face of strong genetic predisposition – confirm that promise.

COLORECTAL CANCER

If you're interested in nutrition, you probably know that the best diet for cancer prevention is one that emphasises whole grains plus fresh fruits and vegetables. No controversy about that. What no one really knows, though, is why it works. Credit usually goes to the antioxidants – chemicals that fight cell damage in our body – that these foods contain. And it's generally assumed that their fibre helps the intestines to clear away carcinogens.

My theory – and I'll tell you about research on colorectal cancer that lends it support – is that our microflora deserves some thanks, too. I think it's no coincidence that the pro-microflora dietary suggestions in this book just happen to be very similar to the anti-cancer diet. When we support our microflora, they return the favour.

Colorectal Cancer Risk Factors

Population studies give us an excellent idea of the factors associated with colorectal cancer. These include age (most people who get this disease are over the age of 50), family history, obesity, inactivity and heavy use of alcohol. But I want to draw your attention to two other important factors on the list: diet and inflammation. Both have microflora connections.

Diet

Scary, but true: all of us eat carcinogens every day. Not only that, our body actually creates carcinogens as it digests high-protein foods such as meat. Experts estimate that diet contributes to a significant fraction of all cancers in the United Kingdom – and it may be higher for colorectal cancer.

Fortunately, our microflora provides some protection. Probiotics secrete certain chemicals that counter carcinogens directly. They also support bacteria in our digestive tract that can break down carcinogens, turning them into various nutrients and harmless molecules. Some of these anti-cancer bacteria are in the 'sometimes good, sometimes bad' category I described in Chapter 2. In other words, they can have harmful effects if they aren't controlled. Someday, we may use them therapeutically. But if we do, it will be done under supervision by a healthcare professional, much as prescription drugs are used today.

The protective activities of our microflora could help to explain why antioxidants fight cancer. Most antioxidants are dietary phenols – prebiotics that help to support probiotics. In addition to their direct effects against cancer, these compounds also may work indirectly, via their positive impact on our microbial population. This is explained further in Chapter 12, about prebiotics.

Fibre is credited with an anti-cancer role, too. Some of this, we assume, is purely mechanical: fibre helps to move wastes through the digestive tract, thereby minimising the opportunity for carcinogens to do their damage. But it may have a microbiological effect as well. Animal studies have shown that fibre supports the growth of microbes that break down carcinogens; these same fibre-supported microbes also make chemicals that help our colon cells resist the damage that could lead to cancer.

Inflammation

Inflammation appears to be a predisposing factor in colorectal cancer. No one is sure why, but the risk of this disease is increased by a history of inflammatory bowel disease. Furthermore, people who regularly take anti-inflammatory drugs, such as aspirin, have decreased risk.

➤ A DIFFERENT KIND OF ◄ SMOKING-CANCER CONNECTION

I'm sure you're aware that smoking causes lung cancer and other respiratory cancers. But you might be surprised to learn that smokers are at elevated risk for colorectal cancer, too. What's more, smoking is linked to cancer of the bladder, cervix, kidneys, pancreas and stomach.

Here's a connection that almost no one thinks about: all the carcinogens that enter your lungs via cigarette smoke also end up in your GI tract. Remember that everything you inhale, you also swallow. So far, I haven't seen any research on the relationship between smoking and the microflora. But I bet that when such studies are performed, they'll show a connection. And that could help to explain why the impact of smoking falls so heavily upon the digestive system.

As Chapter 4 explained, probiotics can help to reduce inflammation in the GI tract. I've also told you about research showing that probiotics can help to prevent and treat inflammatory bowel disease. All this suggests that they might play a role in preventing the inflammation that can lead to colorectal cancer.

The Evidence for Probiotics

In theory, probiotics should help to protect us against colorectal cancer through the various mechanisms described above. But does this really happen in practice? Let me tell you about the evidence we have so far, much of it from animal studies.

These days, scientists can open a laboratory animal supply catalogue and find a remarkable array of 'knockout' mice – genetically engineered mice in which one or more genes are inoperable. Mice bred this way have made-to-order characteristics that are useful for experiments. For example, if certain genes are knocked out, the mice are vulnerable to particular diseases. One type of knockout mouse can't secrete an anti-inflammatory protein called interleukin-10 (IL-10) that mice normally produce. Without this protein to protect them from inflammation, these special mice are at high risk for inflammatory bowel disease and colorectal cancer. If a preventive agent can stop colorectal cancer in IL-10 knockout mice, this indicates a powerful protective effect.

Irish investigators conducted a study with IL-10 knockout mice to see if probiotics could affect their fate. Of the 20 mice in the study, half were given *Lactobacillus* in milk for sixteen weeks; the rest, the control group, drank plain milk. As expected, five of the mice in the control group developed colorectal cancer – a typical rate for IL-10 knockout mice. But this happened to only one of the 10 mice that received the probiotic. Throughout the study, all the mice were checked for signs of intestinal inflammation. Usually, IL-10 mice have this problem because of the protein they lack.

DO ANTIBIOTICS INCREASE BREAST CANCER RISK?

A study showing a connection between antibiotics and breast cancer made headlines in 2004 when it was published in *JAMA*, the *Journal of the American Medical Association*. Researchers compared the pharmacy records and medical histories of 2,266 adult women with breast cancer with those of 7,953 randomly selected women without the disease who were enrolled in the same health plan. The startling finding was that women with breast cancer were more likely to have used antibiotics. Though several subsequent investigations failed to confirm the connection, the possibility is still intriguing. What could explain an association between antibiotics and breast cancer?

Antibiotics affect the microflora, killing some microbes and allowing others to proliferate. If the drugs destroyed the flora that combat carcinogens in the diet and environment but allowed the growth of bacteria that produce carcinogenic compounds – that could explain why breast cancer risk increased.

But sceptics point out that a wide variety of antibiotics all had the same effect in the *JAMA* study, despite the fact that these medications affect different microbes in the microflora. Perhaps, they argue, the women who took antibiotics were generally in poorer health. Or maybe they were taking antibiotics for other conditions that put them at elevated risk for breast cancer.

I can't tell you if antibiotics really increase breast cancer risk. But if they do, that's yet another reason – on top of preventing antibiotic-associated diarrhoea – to take probiotics when these drugs are prescribed.

But there was significantly less inflammation in the probiotics group. These exciting findings – which have been confirmed by other research – were published in *Alimentary Pharmacology and Therapeutics* in 2001.

Of course, it's impossible to conduct such well-controlled research in humans. Even if we could come up with people who had just the right genes, we'd have to persuade them to live in a laboratory, eating only prescribed food, for the years that it takes for humans to develop colorectal cancer. Not very likely!

What to do instead? One approach is to look closely at people who already have the disease, matching them with others who are cancer-free. Then we try to find out what else is different about them. That's one of the ways we learnt about the role of diet and aspirin in preventing colorectal cancer. Yet another kind of human study focuses on cancer markers – signs that show up long before the actual disease. For example, colorectal cancer risk is associated with certain DNA-damaging compounds that can be tracked in human faeces. German investigators demonstrated that these markers were significantly reduced in volunteers after they consumed yoghurt with extra probiotics for six weeks.

As you can see, research strongly suggests that probiotics could be valuable for preventing colorectal cancer. If you're already following an anti-cancer diet in the hope of preventing the disease, you're getting plenty of prebiotics. Adding probiotics won't disrupt your diet. But it could add another potent weapon to the ones you already have.

CARDIOVASCULAR DISEASE

Cholesterol used to get all the blame for cardiovascular disease (CVD). The story went like this: a diet high in saturated fat leads to high levels of cholesterol in the blood. Cholesterol sticks to the arterial walls, narrowing them. If narrowed arteries disrupt blood flow to the heart, the result is a heart attack; if the blockage affects the brain, it produces a stroke. Heart disease and stroke are the most common diseases of the cardiovascular system. CVD is the leading cause of death in the European Union – accounting for over 1.5 million deaths each year.

Studies over the past decade have changed our understanding of CVD. Though cholesterol adds to the risk, an equally significant factor is inflammatory changes in the blood vessels. Without inflammation, high levels of blood cholesterol aren't likely to cause CVD. But even people with apparently healthy cholesterol levels may suffer heart attacks and strokes if their arteries are inflamed.

Whenever I learn that a disease involves inflammation, I always wonder if the microflora might play a part. In the case of CVD, research suggests that it does. If so, there could be a role for probiotics in prevention and treatment.

The Role of Inflammation and White Blood Cells

Scientists now believe that atherosclerosis – the narrowing of blood vessels that leads to heart attacks and strokes – begins when the blood vessels become inflamed. Inflammation can result from injury or damage from an infection.

Are microbes involved in the damage? Maybe. One possible culprit is *Streptococcus mutans*, which causes tooth decay. You may be surprised to learn (as I was when I first heard it) that people who have more cavities are more likely to have heart attacks than those with healthier teeth. However, it's also possible that S. *mutans* or other microbes are innocent bystanders that are targeted by the immune system simply because they happen to be in the neighbourhood.

Whatever the reason for the arterial damage, the tissues call for help. This draws white blood cells to the area, which creates inflammation. We now know that activated phagocytes at the site of arterial inflammation accumulate cholesterol from the blood. If there's a lot of accumulated cholesterol in the phagocytes, or if inflammation continues, the blood vessel may narrow and even close completely.

What could stop the inflammatory process? Regulatory T cells are a prime candidate because of their anti-inflammatory role, which I explained in Chapter 4. These days, they're getting lots of research attention. To me, the combination of microbes, damage, inflammation and regulatory T cells sounds like a job for probiotics!

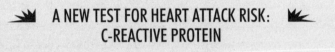

A NEW TEST FOR HEART ATTACK RISK: C-REACTIVE PROTEIN

Inflammation inside the body normally isn't visible. But a simple blood test can spot it. The test measures a molecule called C-reactive protein (CRP), whose presence in the blood indicates inflammation somewhere in the body. Major studies have shown a strong link between a high CRP level and increased risk of heart attack and stroke. Elevated CRP may indeed stem from inflammation in blood vessels. But it also may result from an infection or from a chronic inflammatory condition, such as rheumatoid arthritis.

Preventing CVD with Probiotics

Arterial inflammation and blood cholesterol go hand in hand to create the blockages that cause CVD. Reducing either risk factor helps; reducing both is incredible.

Fighting Inflammation

As Chapter 4 described, probiotics support the development of regulatory T cells, thereby helping to reduce overly exuberant inflammatory responses throughout the body. This remarkable capability has translated into therapeutic use of probiotics for certain inflammatory conditions, such as inflammatory bowel disease. In a sense, CVD might be called 'inflammatory artery disease'. Though there haven't yet been any trials that focus on probiotics for CVD, I feel optimistic about their prospects for addressing that problem, too.

Countering Cholesterol

Studies with laboratory animals consistently show that probiotics can reduce blood cholesterol levels. So far, though, findings in humans have been mixed. Why the difference? It's difficult to control all the relevant variables in humans, such as genetics, diet, exercise and overall health. That's not a problem with lab mice. But I view the animal investigations as feasibility studies. They ask the question, is it at least *possible* that probiotics could lower cholesterol? And the answer is clear: yes.

Here are three possible mechanisms by which probiotic microbes might lower blood cholesterol. Probiotics may:

• **Create acids that counter cholesterol production.** As probiotic bacteria digest soluble fibre in the lower intestines, they produce acids. One of these acids, called propionic acid, decreases synthesis of cholesterol by the liver. That's very much how cholesterol-lowering statin drugs work (e.g. Lipitor, Mevacor, Zocor and many others). When the liver makes less cholesterol, there's less to circulate in the blood.

• **Break down bile acids.** Some probiotic bacteria can break down bile acids. These acids play an important role in fat digestion. They're made from cholesterol by the liver, which dumps them into the intestinal tract. Normally, the liver reabsorbs any excess acids from the intestines and recycles them, so they can be reused for a later meal. But if the acids are broken down by bacteria in the intestines, the liver can't recycle them. So it must draw upon cholesterol in the blood to produce more.

• **Use cholesterol as food.** At least in a laboratory dish, probiotic bacteria can break down cholesterol and use it for their growth. However, it's not yet clear whether this actually happens in the intestines.

I fully expect that human studies will eventually tell us more about using probiotics to lower cholesterol. Particular probiotics might be required, or the results might be affected by variables such as being overweight, smoking and diet.

Meanwhile, human research already shows that soluble fibre – a prebiotic – is linked to lower cholesterol. And another type of prebiotic, dietary phenols, is correlated with decreased CVD risk. That's why heart-healthy diets not only minimise saturated fat but also call for plenty of fruit and vegetables. I can't help thinking that maybe prebiotics are so helpful against CVD in part because of the probiotics whose growth they encourage.

OBESITY

You've seen this simple equation: if the calories you consume are equal to the calories you burn, your weight will remain the same. In other words, if you want to lose weight, you must either eat less or become more active. That always made sense to me – until I learnt about beef cattle and antibiotics.

Bullocks eat hay, which contains about 455 calories per kilo. A bullock's intestinal cells can't break down hay into substances its body can absorb. Instead, bullocks rely upon microbes in their digestive tracts to do it for them. Anything the microbes can't digest ends up as manure. That kilo of hay, which is worth 455 calories in theory, could turn out to be worth only about 320 calories in practice, because anything that ends up in manure isn't going to fatten the animal.

Agricultural researchers devote a lot of attention to what they call 'feed efficiency' in beef cattle – that is, getting bullocks to put on as much weight as possible from the food they eat. They've discovered that if they change a bullock's microflora by administering low doses of antibiotics – which decreases the number of *lactobacilli* in the gut – the animal can extract about 410 calories from the same amount of hay that provided only 320 calories normally. What works this magic? One possibility is that the bullocks are healthier because the antibiotics prevent certain bacterial diseases. But it's clear that changes in their microflora are also involved in increasing feed efficiency.

We're not cattle. We don't have four stomachs, as bullocks do, and chewing the cud is not part of our digestive process. Most of us aren't trying to gain as much weight as possible from the food we eat – quite the contrary! But learning about feed efficiency in livestock, and the role of the microflora in beefing up cattle, got me wondering. Maybe the human weight equation involves more than calories consumed and calories burnt – maybe there's also an M factor: our microflora. And if antibiotics can make bullocks fat, could probiotics possibly help humans to lose weight? A handful of scientists are working on related questions, and I want to tell you about their findings so far.

Our Metabolic Helpers

Recent evidence suggests that our microflora may play an important role in breaking down the food we eat, creating nutrients our body can use. A team of scientists from the Institute for Genomic Research in Rockville, Maryland, USA, analysed the entire microflora of two healthy human volunteers. They hoped to determine if the microbes in our intestinal tract make digestive enzymes that our own body can't make, and whether these enzymes affect how we metabolise food. The answer – published in *Science* in 2006 – was an overwhelming yes. Researchers found hundreds of relevant enzymes made by the microbes we host. These enzymes help break down complex food particles into simple sugars, fats and amino acids (the building blocks of protein), so that our body can absorb them. Thus the microflora contributes quite a bit to human metabolism, though we're still learning about the specifics.

Research in mice provides confirmation that the microflora is a factor in metabolism. Mice are more relevant than bullocks, because their digestive system works basically the same way that ours does. A fascinating study, led by scientists from Washington University in St Louis, Missouri, USA, compared two groups of genetically identical mice. One group was raised normally. The others were microbe-free, like the mice I described in Chapter 1.

All the mice received the same food. But by the time the two groups were about 8 to 10 weeks old, there was a dramatic difference in their weight. Compared with their microbe-free counterparts, the normal mice were much heavier and had 42 per cent more body fat. Evidently, their microflora was affecting how they metabolised food.

Then the researchers exposed the microbe-free mice to microbes from a healthy mouse. Their digestive tracts quickly developed a normal microflora and the consequences were astonishing. These previously lean mice rapidly gained weight. In just fourteen days, their body fat increased by a remarkable 60 per cent. Even more amazing: the mice were actually eating *less* than they'd eaten when they were microbe-free. But now that they had a microflora to assist with metabolism, their bodies could absorb more nutrients from their food.

When the scientists looked more closely at what was happening in the gut, they learnt that the microbes performed two key functions that affected weight. First, they broke down certain dietary components that the mice's own intestinal tracts couldn't digest. It was as if the mice had been eating from lunch boxes that contained secret compartments with extra food – and now the microbes had opened those compartments. Second, the microbes released chemicals that promoted fat storage in the body. Subsequent studies from the same lab have found intriguing differences in the gut microflora of normal mice and mice that have a genetic defect that makes them obese. The next step: attempting to understand the relevance of their findings to humans.

These investigations show that the microflora contributes to metabolism. However, they *don't* suggest that the best way to lose weight is to sterilise your GI tract! Remember that microbe-free mice are not healthy. Their immune systems function poorly and they have other problems, such as an abnormal sleep-wake cycle.

The Gut Microflora and Weight Control

The United Kingdom has the third highest obesity rate in the world, second only to the United States and Mexico. Particularly troubling is the fact that during the past twenty years, obesity has more than doubled among children and trebled among adolescents. Could probiotics make a dent in this enormous problem?

So far, no studies have addressed that question directly. But the potential is clear from the research I've just described. Investigators can cause weight changes in mice simply by manipulating their microflora. They've demonstrated that weight is not just a matter of calories consumed and calories burnt in physical activity – the gut microflora also belongs in the equation. Even if changes in the microflora had only a minor impact in humans, they could make a significant difference over time. What if tinkering with our gut microbes could make our body absorb just 50 calories less per day? In a year, if nothing else changed, that could add up to a loss of about two kilos.

⮞⮞ TANTALISING FINDINGS ⮜⮜

No one has directly studied the effects of probiotics on weight loss efforts. But probiotics have been involved in dieting studies with a different focus. The results make me hopeful.

Researchers from the University of Tennessee, Knoxville, USA, put 34 obese adults on diets. All of them reduced their daily food intake by 500 calories. But half of the participants included yoghurt in their diet – 170 grams, three times a day – while the rest instead ate a gelatin pudding with the same calorific content. After twelve weeks, everyone had lost weight. But those in the yoghurt group lost almost 30 per cent more. The results were published in the *International Journal of Obesity* in 2005.

Should probiotics get the credit? Perhaps, but it's not clear. The investigators were actually looking at the effects of calcium, which has been found to promote weight loss in some studies. Yoghurt provides both calcium and probiotics. Those who consumed gelatin got neither, which could explain all or part of the difference.

We all know that a diet laden with fat and sugar contributes to obesity. But is it just a matter of calories? These foods also shape the microflora by favouring the growth of harmful microbes. And conversely, many studies have found that diets high in fibre aid weight loss. The assumption has been that it's just a matter of bulk: fibre contains no calories, but it provides something to chew and gives a sense of fullness. So it's easier for people to eat less when they consume high-fibre foods. But fibre also acts as a prebiotic, promoting probiotics in the gut. That also could be a factor in the success of high-fibre diets.

COELIAC DISEASE

Take an allergy to gluten – a protein found in wheat and some other grains – and combine it with autoimmunity, and you have coeliac disease. If a person with this condition consumes a slice of toast, a piece of cake, a plate of pasta or any other food with gluten, it stimulates an immune response that causes inflammation in the small intestine. Chronic inflammation ultimately produces damage, which means that nutrients can't be properly absorbed from food. This can lead to anaemia, unwanted weight loss and osteoporosis; in children, the problem can stunt growth.

At least 125,000 people in the UK have coeliac disease. But many experts believe the incidence is much higher, because the condition is commonly misdiagnosed. And as scientists learn more about coeliac disease, they're discovering reasons to believe that probiotics could be highly effective in preventing or treating it.

Symptoms

People with coeliac disease usually suffer from digestive tract problems such as diarrhoea, abdominal pain and wind. But the condition may also involve a wide range of symptoms with no obvious connection to the intestines. The long list of possibilities affects every part of the body and includes irritability, depression, fatigue, joint pain, muscle cramps, sores inside the mouth, tooth discolouration, and a characteristic skin rash. Some individuals with coeliac disease appear healthy – until they develop signs of malnutrition due to intestinal damage.

Because the symptoms vary so much and are easily confused with those of other conditions, coeliac disease may not be recognised straight away. A 2001 Columbia University survey of 1,612 people with the condition found that their symptoms had been present for an average of eleven years before they were properly diagnosed.

When symptoms suggest the possibility of coeliac disease, diagnosis usually begins with blood tests that can identify certain immune reactions. Confirmation requires examination of an intestinal tissue sample to check for the characteristic damage. The sample is obtained via a long, thin viewing and operating tube called an endoscope, which is inserted into the mouth and snaked down through the digestive tract.

Current Treatment

At the moment, the only treatment for coeliac disease is to eliminate all gluten-containing foods. But it's not easy to follow a gluten-free diet. Coeliac patients must not only avoid all wheat, rye and barley products, but also must be on constant watch for the many foods that contain hidden gluten. These include some sausages and cold meats that use wheat as a filler; soups, sauces and salad dressings whose thickeners contain gluten – and even beer, which is made with malted barley. Non-food items can present a risk, too: gluten is found in some lipsticks and in some medications.

The good news is that for most people this drastic dietary change will alleviate symptoms, allowing intestinal damage to be repaired and preventing further damage from inflammatory reactions in the intestines. For those whose symptoms persist despite a gluten-free diet, various medications are used to address the specific difficulties.

Why Probiotics Might Help

Recent studies suggest that the mucus layer of the intestines in coeliac patients is chemically different from that of healthy people, with different types of sugar in the mucus. The difference favours certain harmful bacteria, which therefore stick more firmly to the intestinal walls of people with coeliac disease. The presence of these bacteria may trigger the problematic inflammatory response.

Probiotics might help to prevent or treat coeliac disease because they produce chemicals that prevent other bacteria from sticking to intestinal cells. They also compete for space on the intestinal wall, crowding out harmful bacteria.

Also relevant could be the yeast *Candida albicans*, whose population in the gut is normally kept under control by probiotic bacteria. If this yeast proliferates, the immune system attacks it. Scientists have learnt that a protein made by this yeast is very similar biochemically to part of the gluten protein. This raises the intriguing possibility that the normal immune response to *Candida* might mistakenly target gluten as well. If it turns out that *Candida* plays a role in the development of coeliac disease, then probiotics – by controlling the yeast population – could help to prevent the problem. Certainly, that would be a lot easier than eliminating gluten.

ORAL HEALTH

The thought may be unappealing, but it's true: billions of microbes live in your mouth. Some are bad guys: bacteria that cause cavities, gum disease and bad breath. But according to preliminary studies, probiotics may serve as microscopic dentists, clearing out the germs that interfere with our oral health.

For example, a study done in Turkey found that subjects who ate yoghurt containing *Bifidobacterium* DN-173 010 once daily had fewer cavity-causing bacteria in their mouths than a control group who ate yoghurt that had been treated to kill all the probiotic bacteria. And Japanese researchers found that consumption of *Lactobacillus reuteri* in yoghurt lowered the numbers of both cavity- and odour-producing bacteria in the mouth.

How can probiotics produce such marvellous results? Microbial competition. The good guys take over the turf, crowding out harmful microbes that lurk on surfaces of the teeth, on the tongue and elsewhere in the mouth. For instance, get rid of the bacteria that produce smelly compounds like hydrogen sulphide, and voilà! No more halitosis.

Manufacturers are already taking note. In the pipeline are probiotic toothpastes, mouthwashes and even a chewing gum that could fight tooth decay.

FIBROMYALGIA AND CHRONIC FATIGUE SYNDROME

Imagine having the flu – exhaustion, severe muscular aches, diarrhoea and more – except that it continues for months rather than days. Brief respites occur, only to be followed by flare-ups that sometimes include baffling new symptoms, like dizziness and a strange sensitivity to odours. Physicians can barely provide a diagnosis, much less a treatment: 'I'm not really sure you have a disease. But I've seen this collection of symptoms before, so let's call it a syndrome. And since you seem unhappy and stressed out, I'll prescribe an antidepressant.'

This is the world of fibromyalgia and chronic fatigue syndrome (CFS), highly debilitating conditions with overlapping symptoms. They have no known cause and no known cure. Surprising as it may sound, a closer look at fibromyalgia and CFS suggests the possibility of microflora connections. The pathway involves the immune system and the nervous system.

Possible Causes

Though we don't know what causes fibromyalgia or chronic fatigue syndrome, patients' medical histories often point to triggering events, such as having a viral or bacterial infection or being diagnosed with another disorder, such as rheumatoid arthritis or lupus. In other words, the body has developed inflammation. What may be happening in fibromyalgia and CFS is that this inflammation never goes away completely. For some unknown reason, the regulatory T cells didn't do their job.

Low-level inflammation can affect the nervous system, leading to increased sensitivity to pain. One theory is that inflammation affects pain-related neurotransmitters. This could explain the mysterious symptoms of these conditions. People experience pain, but there's no obvious physical cause. Perhaps the nervous system is overreacting, experiencing normal muscle contractions and stretches as pain.

One clue in support of that idea comes from the fact that people with fibromyalgia and CFS often suffer from irritable bowel syndrome (IBS) as well. IBS involves such hypersensitivity: individuals with this condition feel pain from stretching of the intestines that most of us experience merely as a pleasant sense of fullness. One study that questioned patients about details of their symptoms found that 77 per cent of those with fibromyalgia and 92 per cent of those with CFS also reported irritable bowel syndrome.

As I explained in Chapter 6, IBS may be caused by a problem called small intestinal bacterial overgrowth (SIBO), in which microbes that normally live in the large intestine overgrow into the small intestine. The result is wind, bloating and pain. It turns out that SIBO also could be a factor in fibromyalgia. California researchers recruited 42 fibromyalgia patients, 111 people with irritable bowel syndrome and 15 controls who had neither condition. All received a test for SIBO that measures hydrogen in the breath (see page 119 for details). Those with fibromyalgia also were asked to rate their pain on a standard scale. Some of the controls – 20 per cent – had the high levels of hydrogen associated with SIBO. But the condition was diagnosed in 84 per cent of those with irritable bowel syndrome and in 100 per cent of people with fibromyalgia! Particularly interesting was that among those with fibromyalgia, the higher their score on the hydrogen test for SIBO, the greater their reported pain.

Could Probiotics Help?

Clinical studies have already shown that probiotics can bring relief to patients with irritable bowel syndrome and SIBO. Given what we know about the links between IBS and fibromyalgia and chronic fatigue, there's excellent reason to believe that probiotics could help treat these conditions as well.

One promising hint comes from animal studies that have found probiotics can reduce the nervous system hypersensitivity involved in fibromyalgia and CFS. Another is that several preliminary investigations have found that fibromyalgia is relieved by a diet of raw foods rich in prebiotics.

In one of these studies, performed in Finland, 18 fibromyalgia patients volunteered to follow a highly restricted diet. The permitted foods included the following, all of which were consumed uncooked: fruit, berries, vegetables, mushrooms, nuts, seeds, legumes and cereals. A control group of 15 patients simply ate as usual. When the study began, the two groups reported similar symptoms. But after three months, there were striking differences: those on the special diet had significantly less pain and stiffness and greatly improved sleep. At the end of the initial study period, participants were allowed to eat as they pleased, but the researchers continued to follow them for another five months. None of the patients in the raw foods group stuck with the diet, despite their improvements. Over the next few months, their fibromyalgia symptoms gradually returned to the previous level. Results were published in the *Scandinavian Journal of Rheumatology* in 2000.

Could changes in the microflora be responsible for the symptom relief seen with the raw food diet? It's possible: a diet high in prebiotics provides support for probiotics in the GI tract. A microflora that contains more probiotics favours the development of regulatory T cells, which can prevent low-level inflammation and the problematic signals it sends to the nervous system.

Though this chain of reasoning is logical, other factors may have been at work. Those who followed the diet lost a significant amount of weight, which probably reduced their aches and pains. And of course, pain is subjective. The ideal way to test probiotics as a treatment for fibromyalgia and CFS would involve a 'blind' study in which participants don't know whether or not they're getting the measure under investigation. But for obvious practical reasons, participants in the Finnish study knew they were in the treatment group. So we can't tell how much credit the placebo effect deserves.

I look forward to more focused clinical trials that continue these promising leads. Perhaps measures similar to those in this book – easy-to-follow dietary recommendations and high-quality probiotic supplements – could help to relieve these physically and emotionally debilitating syndromes, which so far have eluded medical science.

AUTISM

When Andrew Bolte was 17 months old, his paediatrician prescribed a six-week course of antibiotics for chronic ear infections. Andrew developed diarrhoea, a common side effect of antibiotics. Far more alarming: within two months, his previously normal mental and social development regressed. He stopped speaking and would no longer make eye contact with people, even his mother and father. Sometimes he screamed for hours, for no apparent reason. His behaviour became unmanageable. He'd bang his head and claw at anyone who tried to stop him. Andrew's parents were distraught. Their child was deteriorating before their eyes and they didn't know how to stop it. Doctors finally gave them a dire diagnosis: autism.

Autism is a tragic, baffling condition that affects an estimated 500,000 families in the United Kingdom. Though there are various types of autism, some far more disabling than others, all involve deficient social and communication skills, as well as behavioural abnormalities. Parents can usually tell very early in childhood that their child is different. But sometimes, as in Andrew Bolte's case, a child follows a normal developmental path for the first year or two and then veers off.

New Thinking About Autism

Experts agree that autism is caused by brain abnormalities. But the reason (or reasons) for these abnormalities is unknown. Genes may be a factor in some cases – identical twins are far more likely than fraternal twins to share this problem. Other possibilities include exposure to toxins, either in utero or after birth; nutritional deficiencies; and viral or bacterial infections. I've been following one fascinating hypothesis, which involves antibiotics and the gut microflora. This idea was first championed by Ellen Bolte, Andrew's mother.

Desperate to help her son, Bolte studied the medical and scientific literature. She began to wonder if the antibiotics Andrew had received for his ear infections may have killed protective bacteria in his gut, permitting the proliferation of *Clostridium tetani*. This dangerous bacterium produces a potent neurotoxin that disrupts chemical signals in the brain. Previous research, she learnt, had shown that the neurotoxin could create autistic-like behavioural changes in animals. Moreover, there was evidence that some children with autism had improved when given antibiotics that can kill *Clostridium*.

Bolte approached several doctors with her theory. Most were sceptical. But a physician at Rush Children's Hospital in Chicago, Illinois, USA, Richard Sandler, agreed to treat her son with vancomycin, a powerful antibiotic known to be effective against *Clostridium*. To Dr Sandler's surprise, the child improved dramatically. Tragically, with the end of treatment came the loss of most of the boy's gains.

To further test Ellen Bolte's hypothesis, and to confirm the effects of vancomycin, Dr Sandler undertook a study of 11 children, including Andrew, whose autism developed after antibiotic therapy followed by persistent diarrhoea. Treatment with vancomycin produced significant short-term improvements in eight of the children studied. But as before, these encouraging changes were short-lived.

Treating Autism with Probiotics

Vancomycin and other antibiotics are not a feasible long-term treatment for autism, because the bacteria will inevitably become resistant to the drugs. And in any case, long-term use of antibiotics can have other adverse consequences for health. Moreover, not all autistic children have the medical history – antibiotics followed by diarrhoea and regression – that's characteristic of those helped by vancomycin. But the insights gained by this research have sparked interest in other treatment approaches.

Investigators at the University of Reading are attempting to learn if probiotic food supplements might reduce symptoms in autistic children. The idea is to use probiotics to decrease the number of *Clostridium* through microbial competition. According to news reports, initial results have been both frustrating and extremely encouraging.

The scientists recruited 40 autistic children aged 4 to 8. In the first stage of the study, half received a powdered supplement containing the probiotic *Lactobacillus plantarum*; the others were given a placebo powder. Parents were asked to administer the powder daily and to record their child's autistic symptoms in a diary. The plan for the second stage of the study was to swap treatments, so that each child would have a period on both the probiotic and the placebo.

To avoid biasing the diaries, parents were not told which powder they were using. But during stage one – as parents kept track of their child's mood, level of concentration and behaviour – those assigned to the probiotic group figured it out. Improvements were so striking that when the time came to switch groups, these parents refused. There were so many dropouts that the experiment was declared a 'failure'. But because of the obvious success of probiotic treatment, the researchers have promised additional studies.

Unlike antibiotics, the supplements have no adverse side effects. If probiotics work, they can be continued for as long as necessary. And since probiotic foods and supplements are safe, there's no need to wait for conclusive scientific evidence. Note, however, that even the most enthusiastic advocates of probiotic treatment don't claim that it can help all autistic children.

Some people despair of finding cures for chronic diseases like cancer and the other conditions discussed in this chapter. They throw up their hands and say, 'This is much too complex for a simple answer.' But I'm an optimist by nature. My reaction is to say, 'Maybe we're overlooking something big – a new idea? a new concept?'

Could microflora theory and probiotic therapy be a break-through for these problems? Yes. Only time and well-designed clinical studies will provide the definitive answers. But in the interim, you can easily – and safely – incorporate probiotics into your diet. Will you see positive changes if you suffer from a chronic disease? I can't promise that you will. But I hope you feel as optimistic as I do.

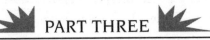

PART THREE

Promoting Microbial Balance: What You Can Do

Let food be thy medicine and medicine be thy food.

– HIPPOCRATES

CHAPTER TEN

Food Sources of Probiotics

Centuries ago, before the invention of refrigeration, people used other methods – such as cooking and salting – to extend the life of food. Fermentation is another ancient preservation technique: bacteria break down nutrients, turning them into chemicals that help to keep food from deteriorating. Examples of fermentation include transforming milk into yoghurt and cheese, pickling cucumbers and other vegetables and turning cabbage into sauerkraut.

You can see from these examples that fermentation doesn't just preserve; it also changes flavour and texture. In addition, as we're now learning, fermentation actually enriches food, adding health-promoting probiotics. This chapter describes delicious foods that put these beneficial microbes to work for you. Some will be familiar; others may be new.

FERMENTING FOR FLAVOUR AND HEALTH

The bacteria used for fermentation – many of them probiotics – live naturally in milk and on the surfaces of grains, vegetables and fruit. They're called lactic acid bacteria because during fermentation, they produce lactic acid as well as other chemicals that counter the bacteria responsible for spoilage. Lactic acid also accounts for the tart flavour that characterises fermented foods.

The health benefits of fermentation come from two sources. First, probiotic bacteria proliferate as food ferments. When we eat foods that contain live probiotics, we're delivering an army to our digestive tract – friendly warriors that will do battle against harmful microbes and boost our immune system. Fermented foods also contain what I call 'metabiotics', helpful metabolic by-products from the bacteria. When probiotic bacteria digest fibre and other nutrients, they produce waste products that are actually beneficial to our health.

In addition, many fermented foods are a source of prebiotics – compounds that make the digestive tract more hospitable to probiotic microbes. One example is lactoferrin, a protein found in whey (the liquid part of curdled milk) that has antimicrobial properties. Lactoferrin is contained in yoghurt and in other fermented dairy products that include whey. Other examples of prebiotics in fermented foods are the fibre and antioxidants in pickled vegetables. You'll hear more about prebiotics in Chapter 12.

Probiotic bacteria are living organisms. If they're exposed to heat or other adverse conditions, they will die. In contrast, prebiotics and metabiotics are usually more stable under adverse conditions. For instance, if you add yoghurt to a sauce and simmer it, the probiotic bacteria will not survive – but the prebiotics and metabiotics will remain.

HOW MUCH DO I NEED?

I'm convinced that someday we'll have research-based minimum daily requirements for probiotics, just as we do for many vitamins and minerals. In the meantime, we can make approximations based on the collective experience of scientists who study these beneficial microbes. Such educated guesses match what we know about healthy populations whose diets are rich in probiotics – including the Bulgarian peasants Ilya Mechnikov studied decades ago.

To come up with the recommendations in this chapter, I compiled information on the quantities scientists use in published peer-reviewed research about probiotic foods and health. We can feel confident that these amounts are safe and effective. In the future, as our collective knowledge is refined, we'll be able to optimise these recommendations. Also, I'm hopeful that probiotic labelling will improve. At the moment, the exact probiotic content of foods isn't described on their labels – and indeed, it's sometimes untested and unknown. At best, the label indicates how many bacteria were present at the time of manufacture.

The table below shows the approximate probiotic content of the foods discussed in this chapter, when available; I've also estimated their prebiotic and metabiotic content. For convenience in daily menu planning, I've used the term 'probiotic serving unit' for a food portion that contains about 3 to 10 billion bacteria at the time of manufacture. Here are my suggestions:

FOOD SOURCES OF PROBIOTICS

(Probiotic serving unit = approximately 3 to 10 billion bacteria
at the time of manufacture)

FOOD AND SPECIES OR STRAINS CONTAINED	PORTION SIZE	PROBIOTIC SERVING UNITS PER PORTION	METABIOTIC CONTENT	PREBIOTIC CONTENT
Yoghurt with live bacteria *Lactobacillus bulgaricus; Streptococcus thermophilus;* others may be added — check label	170 to 230 grams	1 to 2	High	Low; medium if it contains added fibre
Yoghurt without live bacteria; yoghurt used in cooking No probiotics	170 to 230 grams	None	High	Low; medium if it contains added fibre
Frozen yoghurt with live bacteria *Lactobacillus bulgaricus; Streptococcus thermophilus*	110 grams	¼	Low	Negligible
Probiotic 'shots' — milk drinks and yoghurt Various strains; see label	85 to 110 grams	1 to 2	Medium to high	Low
Aged cheese *Lactobacillus* strains and others, depending on type of cheese	45 grams	1	High	Negligible

FOOD AND SPECIES OR STRAINS CONTAINED	PORTION SIZE	PROBIOTIC SERVING UNITS PER PORTION	METABIOTIC CONTENT	PREBIOTIC CONTENT
Kefir Usually contains *Lactobacillus*, *Bifidobacterium* and many others – check label	240 ml	1	High	Low to medium (if contains added fibre)
Other cultured dairy products *Lactobacillus acidophilus* in acidophilus milk; *Lactococcus lactis* and *Leuconostoc* in buttermilk and soured cream; others may be added as enrichment to other dairy foods such as cottage cheese	120 to 240 ml	Negligible; low to high if product is enriched with probiotics	Low	Low
Other fermented foods (pickles, sauerkraut, kimchi, miso soup) *Lactobacillus* and other lactic acid bacteria	Various	Unknown, but probably ranges from low to high	High	High

• If you're healthy, aim for at least one or two probiotic serving units daily.

• If you're hoping to prevent or address medical problems, consume two or three units per day.

• Select foods that contain a variety of probiotics. In particular, try to include both *Lactobacillus* and *Bifidobacterium* bacteria.

YOGHURT

Ever since Nobel laureate Ilya Mechnikov studied the remarkable longevity of Bulgarian peasants, yoghurt has been credited with promoting health. To this day, yoghurt is made from the same bacterial species, *Lactobacillus bulgaricus*, which Mechnikov isolated a century ago from the fermented foods he discovered in Bulgaria. Though other readily available foods contain probiotics, yoghurt remains the premier source of these beneficial bacteria. Like other dairy products, yoghurt is an excellent source of protein and calcium, too.

Food historians speculate that yoghurt was first made accidentally, when milk was left inside goatskin bags and fermented by wild bacteria. These days, most yoghurts are commercially manufactured by a process that's considerably less spontaneous. The milk, which can come from any milk-producing animal, is first pasteurised (i.e., heated sufficiently to kill any harmful bacteria), and then bacterial cultures are added to ferment it. These cultures, containing *Lactobacillus bulgaricus* and *Streptococcus thermophilus* are often referred to as yoghurt starters.

The starter bacteria digest lactose (milk sugar) and other carbohydrates in the milk, producing lactic acid and other acids that give yoghurt its characteristic tart taste. The acids also react chemically with milk proteins, causing the milk to thicken. In addition, since harmful bacteria can't grow in an acidic environment, the acids protect the milk from contamination. On top of these useful effects are all the health benefits from probiotic bacteria and from metabiotics, the metabolic products that probiotic bacteria produce. Yoghurt also contains lactoferrin, a prebiotic found in milk.

After fermentation, fruit, jam or other flavourings may be added or blended into the yoghurt. Some manufacturers add fibre, which boosts the prebiotic content.

Selecting a Yoghurt

These days, the yoghurt section of a typical supermarket contains dozens of options. In addition to the familiar pots of spoonable yoghurt, there's yoghurt that's sipped and yoghurt in tubes to be squeezed into your mouth. But not all of these yoghurts are created equal for health. Here's how to pick one that will deliver the benefits of probiotics – without empty sugar calories or excess fat.

Look for Probiotics

The best way to ensure that you're buying a yoghurt that contains probiotics is to select a product with a 'live and active cultures' label. Some yoghurts with live bacteria may read 'Contains active yoghurt cultures' or 'Contains living yoghurt cultures'. But avoid yoghurts that simply say 'Made with active cultures'. Such a yoghurt may have been heat-treated after fermentation, in which case the bacteria would no longer be alive.

All yoghurts with live bacteria contain the starters *Lactobacillus bulgaricus* and *Streptococcus thermophilus*. However, some manufacturers add other bacteria to their yoghurts, including the probiotics *L. acidophilus*, *Bifidobacterium animalis*, *L. casei*, *L. reuteri* and others. Check the label.

I recommend 'live and active cultures' yoghurts, but if you can find a brand that includes additional probiotics, that's even better. Research indicates that different probiotic microbes provide different benefits; some are more potent than others. But we don't yet know the full range of effects for each species or strain available in food. So the best way to maximise health benefits is to consume a variety. Since all yoghurts with live bacteria contain *Lactobacillus*, try to find one that also provides bacteria from the *Bifidobacterium* family.

Check the Expiry Date

Probiotic bacteria usually can survive for three to five weeks in refrigerated yoghurt. But check the expiry date and consume the yoghurt promptly so you get the maximum benefit. One reassurance: while it's important to store your yoghurt supply in the refrigerator, keeping a container at room temperature for a lunch or snack to be consumed later that day will not cause any significant loss in probiotic activity.

Watch Out for Sugar

Though plain yoghurt tastes tart, it contains lactose, the sugar that's naturally found in milk. Sugar and sugar-laden fruit preserves often are added to give yoghurt more taste appeal. The total amount of sugar in sweetened yoghurt – natural plus added – may surprise you: it's even more than in a glass of fizzy drink. Of course, yoghurt offers much more nutritional benefit than fizzy drinks and many other sweets.

You can easily determine how much sugar is found in a pot of yoghurt – just read the label. Not quite so simple is learning to enjoy yoghurt that's less sweet.

When I started my probiotic food plan, I couldn't imagine eating plain yoghurt. Nature has given us an attraction to sweet things, and food producers cater to this attraction by adding large amounts of sugar to lots of foods. The more sugar we consume, the more we need to make food taste appealing. But I knew that if I added sweetened yoghurt to my diet, I'd be consuming more sugar than would be healthy for me. So I decided to retrain my taste buds to appreciate tart and sour flavours. The key, I found, was gradual change. After about six months, I was enjoying plain yoghurt. Some tips for making the transition:

• Mix gradually increasing amounts of plain yoghurt into your sweetened yoghurt.
• Instead of buying fruit-on-the-bottom yoghurt, add a small

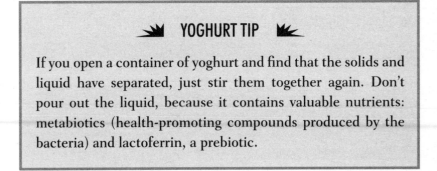

amount of fruit preserves or fruit spread to plain yoghurt. Select preserves that contain less sugar and more fruit.

• Sweeten plain yoghurt with fruit, such as fresh or frozen berries. Bonus: fruit contributes fibre, antioxidants and other prebiotics.

• Swirl a spoonful of honey into plain yoghurt – not just for sweetness and flavour, but also because honey may be a prebiotic.

• Add the distraction of crunch with muesli or cereal. Read the labels to select nutritious products that provide fibre without excess fat, sugar and sodium.

YOGHURT TIP

If you open a container of yoghurt and find that the solids and liquid have separated, just stir them together again. Don't pour out the liquid, because it contains valuable nutrients: metabiotics (health-promoting compounds produced by the bacteria) and lactoferrin, a prebiotic.

Consider the Fat Content

Regular milk – and yoghurt made from it – contains saturated fat. Doctors and nutritionists recommend that adults limit their consumption of saturated fat, not only to protect their cardiovascular system but also to control their weight: the higher the fat content of the yoghurt, the more calories it contains.

Health concerns have prompted yoghurt manufacturers to offer reduced-fat versions. Here's what the labels mean:

• Regular yoghurt: made from whole or full-fat milk (greater than 3 per cent milk fat)

• Low-fat yoghurt: made from low-fat or semi-skimmed milk (between 0.5 per cent and 2 per cent milk fat)

- Non-fat yoghurt: made from skimmed milk (less than 0.5 per cent milk fat)
- Light or lite yoghurt (usually refers to yoghurt sweetened with an artificial sweetener): contains one-third the calories compared with regular yoghurt.

My own preference is for low-fat yoghurt. I like to minimise my intake of saturated fat, but I find that a small amount gives yoghurt an appealing creamy taste. If you eat regular yoghurt, limit other fat consumption so that the total is not excessive.

Get the Bonus of Added Fibre

We don't normally think of dairy foods as sources of fibre – after all, there's no fibre in milk. But some yoghurt manufacturers add fibre to their yoghurt. That's good news, because fibre provides nutritional benefits and extra prebiotics. So look for this bonus ingredient on the label. It usually comes in one of these three forms:

- Pectin, a type of fibre found in apples. Pectin serves double duty. First, it helps to prevent the yoghurt from separating. Second, it acts as a prebiotic, promoting the health of probiotic bacteria.
- Inulin, a fibre that's found in a great many fruit and vegetables.
- FOS (fructo-oligosaccharide), another fibre that's similar to inulin.

Like pectin, inulin and FOS are prebiotics. However, they're considered 'super prebiotic fibres' compared with pectin and the fibre found in wholewheat, because they're significantly better at fostering probiotic growth in the intestinal tract.

➤ WHAT ABOUT MAKING YOGHURT AT HOME? ➤

Home-made yoghurt is a healthy food — as proven by the peasants whom Mechnikov studied. And a family yoghurt-making session might entice children who've been reluctant to eat it. If you're interested in giving home-made yoghurt a try, look for articles on the Internet that explain how it's done. You'll discover many recipes, as well as a wide variety of electric appliances that make the process simple.

To maximise health benefits, choose a starter that contains not only the standard *Lactobacillus bulgaricus* and *Streptococcus thermophilus*, but also a variety of other probiotic bacteria. Yoghurt starters can be purchased at some health food stores or online. Or simply use a small amount of a commercial yoghurt with live bacteria. You could even experiment by adding probiotics from supplements to the yoghurt starters — just open a capsule or packet of one of the supplements recommended in Chapter 11, and stir in the powder.

⚔ PROBIOTIC 'SHOTS' ⚔

Probiotic 'shots' have a long history, although their popularity has had a recent surge. Simply, they are mini servings of probiotic-enriched sweetened milk drinks and yoghurt. Typically, they're sold as single bottles or pots containing just a small amount. Because portions are small, these products are sometimes called 'shots'. A few examples:

• **Actimel**: A cultured milk drink that contains yoghurt starters plus *Lactobacillus casei* DN-114 001 (trade name *L. casei* Defensis or *L. casei* Immunitas), with a total of more than 10 billion bacteria in a 100 ml bottle. Actimel is sweetened and comes in several flavours.

• **Yakult**: A Japanese cultured milk drink with the probiotic *Lactobacillus casei* Shirota. Yakult's 65 ml bottles contain 6.5 billion bacteria. The drink is sweetened and flavoured.

• **Activia**: Sweetened yoghurt, sold in 120 ml pots in a choice of flavours. Activia contains yoghurt starters plus 10 billion *Bifidobacterium animalis* DN-173 010 (trade name: *Bifidus Regularis*).

Though probiotic shots are sold as food – you'll find them in the dairy section at many supermarkets – they're more like supplements in function (and in price). The three products listed above contain bacterial strains that have been scientifically tested for effective probiotic activity. Check the labels for shots as you would for supplements; see Chapter 11 for more information about selecting a probiotic supplement.

Other Yoghurt Products

You'll find other yoghurt – or yoghurt-like – products in the supermarket. Some contain probiotics, but others don't.

Frozen Yoghurt

Beneficial bacteria can survive freezing. So in theory at least, frozen yoghurt can contain probiotics. But in practice, few commercial frozen yoghurts do: yoghurt usually is heated during the manufacturing process, and that's fatal to the bacteria (though it doesn't destroy any metabiotics or prebiotics). Two suggestions if you enjoy frozen yoghurt – but would like it even more with probiotics:

- Look for brands that say 'Contains live and active cultures'. Realise, however, that frozen yoghurt meets a more lenient standard than regular yoghurt, namely 10 million lactic acid bacteria per gram at the time of manufacture instead of more than 100 million per gram. Since a typical serving is only 120 ml, this translates to about 1 billion live bacteria per portion compared with more than 20 billion for a full cup of plain yoghurt.
- Make your own frozen yoghurt. Add flavourings to probiotic-containing yoghurt and then freeze it. One option is to use an ice cream maker, which chills and stirs the mixture. Another is simply to freeze the yoghurt and then blend it in a blender or food processor to achieve the desired texture. Chapter 16 contains a few recipes for home-made frozen yoghurt.

Soya 'Yoghurt'

This yoghurt lookalike isn't really yoghurt, because it's a non-dairy product made from soya milk. But it's prepared the same way, using the same bacterial starters as regular yoghurt. Manufacturers of soya yoghurt often enhance its probiotic content with additional bacteria. Like dairy yoghurt, it contains metabiotics. And because it's soya-based, it also offers fibre, a prebiotic.

Soya yoghurt is an excellent probiotic option, especially for vegans or anyone who can't tolerate dairy foods. If you can't find it in your local supermarket, try a health food store. Check the label as you would for any other yoghurt.

Yoghurt-Covered Snacks

Yoghurt-covered snacks – such as nuts, dried fruit and cereal bars – are popular. But alas, they offer no probiotic value. The yoghurt covering actually contains more sugar than yoghurt. Moreover, it's baked, which kills the bacteria. If you enjoy these snacks, consider them sugar-coated treats and consume accordingly.

KEFIR

When I first started using probiotics, my main food sources were yoghurt and cheese. After about eight months, I decided to explore other options. Mairi Noverr suggested I try kefir (pronounced either 'kuh-FEAR' or 'KEH-fur'), a fermented milk drink. She'd heard about it from a friend, tried it and liked it. At the time, my local supermarket didn't carry kefir (though it does now). But I found it at a health food store. I was pleased to see that the label promised ten different probiotic microbes, and that the flavoured versions contained less sugar than most flavoured yoghurts. I bought a bottle of plain kefir and a bottle of strawberry – and liked them both.

As Mairi promised, kefir has the tartness of yoghurt, though the flavour is different. That's not surprising, since different microbes are used to manufacture it. When you first open a bottle of kefir, it may be too thick to pour. But if you shake the bottle vigorously before you open it, the kefir will have the creamy consistency of a milkshake – and it will maintain that consistency even if it's stored in the refrigerator for several days. Kefir is now a regular part of my family's menu of probiotic-rich foods. It's a great instant breakfast for mornings when we're running late, and makes an easy mid-afternoon snack. My children love flavoured kefir as a drink to accompany dinner.

The health benefits of kefir have been touted for centuries. However, there's very little published scientific research about it. But since we know that kefir is a fermented milk product, we can assume it contains all the beneficial nutrients found in milk, along with those derived from fermentation and live probiotics.

Unlike yoghurt, which always includes two particular starter bacteria, kefir can be prepared from any of more than two dozen different starter cultures. These cultures, called 'kefir grains', include many varieties of lactic acid bacteria and sometimes a probiotic species of the yeast *Saccharomyces*. Kefir manufacturers don't have a strict standard for microbial content. However, individual producers may provide this information on the label or on their website.

In general, the bacteria count in kefir is lower than in most yoghurts with live cultures. However, kefir offers more diversity of probiotics. I consider a serving of kefir to be roughly equivalent to that of a serving of yoghurt when planning my daily probiotic intake. To optimise microbial counts and variety of probiotics, I consume both kefir and yoghurt regularly. If you've never tasted kefir, I urge you to give it a try. The more probiotic options you have, the better – not only to diversify your gut microflora but to keep your taste buds happy.

WHAT ABOUT ACIDOPHILUS MILK, BUTTERMILK AND SOURED CREAM?

Lactic acid bacteria are used to make acidophilus milk, buttermilk and soured cream. But at the moment, these foods usually aren't useful sources of probiotics: the number of live bacteria they contain – if any remain after processing – is only a small fraction of what's found in yoghurt and kefir. However, that is starting to change. Some manufacturers have already begun to boost the probiotic content of these and other dairy products. But so far, we don't have as much specific information as we do for many yoghurts about the strains and the number of bacteria they contain.

CHEESE

Cheese is made from the milk of cows, goats, sheep, buffalo and other domesticated animals. Sometimes the milk is coagulated with acid or enzymes. But the vast majority of cheeses are produced by fermentation. Like yoghurt and kefir, fermented cheeses – Cheddar, Swiss, parmesan, gouda and hundreds of others – contain live microbes and their health-promoting metabolic products.

Production of fermented cheeses begins with a starter culture of lactic acid bacteria. Different ones are used to make different types of cheese. The bacteria produce lactic acid during fermentation, causing the milk to form curds. Sometimes other ingredients – including additional microbes – are added. Curds are strained from the remaining liquid (whey) and drained. The resulting cheese is allowed to age and ferment for periods ranging from a few days to months or even years; this process is also called 'ripening'. As the cheese ripens, probiotic bacteria produce chemicals that give cheese its distinctive flavour, inhibit spoilage and also create health benefits.

Fermented cheese contains live probiotics. I wish I could tell you how much, but we don't know. Probably it varies by the type of cheese and length of ageing, among other variables. While cheese doesn't have significant prebiotic content – that's because the whey is drained off – it's rich in metabiotics. The longer a cheese has aged, the more of these valuable metabolic products it accumulates. And regardless of age, cheese is a useful source of calcium and protein.

A Healthy Amount of Cheese

Current guidelines for healthy eating usually warn that cheese is high in calories and high in saturated fat; they advise eating cheese only in strictly limited quantities. I think these guidelines need to be revised. At the moment, most mainstream nutritionists don't even consider the probiotic and metabiotic content of cheese. So of course it looks like a hunk of fat that contains calcium. Unfortunately, such thinking sells the nutritional value of cheese short. And I'm pleased that some in the nutrition community are beginning to agree.

No matter how you slice it, there's room for fermented cheeses in a healthy diet. Let's do the maths. About 50 grams of cheese, such as cheddar, contains about 170 calories. That's not difficult to incorporate into an average 2,000-calorie diet. Standard guidelines suggest that no more than 30 per cent of daily caloric intake come from fat – in other words, 600 of those 2,000 calories. Fifty grams of cheese contains about 125 fat calories, no more than a quarter of the recommended limit.

Health studies that show an association between cardiac risk and saturated fat have focused on the total amount consumed, without considering the source. However, several recent reports suggest that the fat in cheese is not as detrimental to the body as the saturated fat in milk or butter. For example, Danish researchers put 14 research subjects on three different diets, respectively featuring generous quantities of whole or full-fat milk, butter or cheddar cheese. Participants remained on each diet for three weeks, and then received tests to measure the fat in their blood.

Not surprisingly, blood cholesterol levels rose following the periods of high whole milk and butter consumption. But cholesterol actually dropped slightly after three weeks of a diet that included nearly 60 grams of cheddar per day. Why the difference? No one is sure. The investigators mentioned two possibilities: the relatively high calcium content of cheese and the fact that it's fermented. Their findings were published in the *Journal of the American College of Nutrition* in 2004.

While most research has focused on the probiotic potential of individual species and strains of *Lactobacillus* and *Bifidobacterium*, one of the lactic acid bacteria used to make cheese has begun to make its way into the probiotic supplement arena: *Propionibacterium*. This bacterium – along with *Streptococcus thermophilus* and *Lactobacillus* – is used to make the type of Swiss cheese called Emmental. It's the most common cheese produced in France and is also made in Switzerland, Finland and Germany. A 50 gram slice contains almost 40 billion live *Propionibacteria*. Research has shown that this probiotic can promote a healthy colon microflora. One of its effects is to help our own *Bifidobacteria* grow to higher numbers. Increasing numbers of studies – including projects in my own laboratory – are investigating the probiotic activities of bacteria in aged cheeses. As a cheese lover, I'm particularly looking forward to clinical findings about the health benefits of these bacteria.

THE MEDITERRANEAN DIET: DO PROBIOTICS EXPLAIN ITS SUCCESS?

Experts concerned about the high incidence of heart disease have wondered what lessons might be learnt from the diets of people who live in Greece, Italy, France and other countries that border the Mediterranean Sea. Inhabitants of Mediterranean countries consume a diet that's relatively high in fat – yet their hearts are healthier than ours.

There's no single Mediterranean diet; specifics vary from country to country. But the common features include abundant fresh fruit and vegetables, as well as whole grains. Also, most of the dairy consumption involves cheese or yoghurt. My guess is that this diet owes its success at least in part to probiotics, prebiotics and metabiotics.

Other Cheeses

Not all cheeses provide probiotic benefits. As I mentioned above, some cheeses aren't fermented; instead, milk or whey is coagulated with an acid or enzyme. The resulting cheeses contain no probiotics or metabiotics, though they all provide calcium and may contain lactoferrin if whey is used.

Mozzarella

Sometimes mozzarella is prepared with acid or enzymes, so it's not fermented. Unless the label lists 'cheese cultures', don't assume it contains probiotics.

Cottage Cheese

Cottage cheese may be cultured with lactic acid bacteria, but not necessarily; sometimes acid or enzymes are used. A few manufacturers have begun to add probiotics to cottage cheese – a practice that I expect to become more common. At the moment, they don't state the amount of live bacteria per serving in these products; nor are there industry standards. But I hope this will change as the public becomes aware of the health benefits of probiotics. Meanwhile, look for brands that contain added bacteria, such as *Lactobacillus acidophilus*. You may notice that cultured cottage cheese tastes tarter than cottage cheese made with acid or enzymes. That's because the bacteria have consumed some of the milk's natural sugar.

Ricotta

Most cheese is prepared from whole or skimmed milk – but ricotta is made from whey, the liquid that's left after curds are removed during cheese making. Thanks to the whey, ricotta contains the prebiotic lactoferrin. However, it has no probiotics or metabiotics, because curds are formed by reheating the whey (*ricotta* means 'recooked' in Italian), and not by fermentation.

Processed Cheese

Processed cheeses aren't really cheese. They're made from real cheese that's been aged briefly. During processing – which is designed to give these products a smooth, creamy texture, even when melted – the cheese is heated and emulsifiers are added. Heat kills the bacterial starters; the emulsifiers destroy the metabiotics produced during the cheese's brief ageing. Thus, processed cheese lacks most of the nutritional benefits of cheese, while retaining all of the fat. My advice: stick with the real thing.

Maximising the Benefits of Cheese

We know much less about the probiotic content of cheeses than we know about the bacteria in yoghurt and kefir. Most manufacturers don't promote cheese as a source of probiotics. I expect this to change as consumer interest in probiotics grows.

In the meantime, here are some general suggestions:

• Choose fermented cheeses. Those made without a bacterial culture don't contain probiotics or metabiotics.
• Select aged cheeses. The longer the cheese ages, the more probiotics and metabiotics it contains.
• Vary your cheese choices. Different cheeses are made with different bacterial cultures, and we don't yet know which particular bacteria provide the most benefits.
• To retain the probiotic value of cheese, don't heat it above 38°C. However, even cooked or melted cheese provides metabiotics.
• Keep a lookout for the healthier cheeses of the future, including cheeses produced from milk with added omega-3 fatty acids.

OTHER FERMENTED FOODS

Many types of fermented foods are consumed throughout the world, including products made from vegetables, fruit and grains. Though health-promoting properties have been ascribed to them through the ages, we know much less about their probiotic content than we know about that of fermented dairy products. Until we have more information, I wouldn't suggest that you make these foods the mainstay of your probiotic eating plan. But why not give them a try?

WHAT IF I'M LACTOSE INTOLERANT?

Lactose intolerance is an inability to digest lactose, the predominant sugar in milk and other dairy products. Symptoms – which generally start an hour or so after eating or drinking lactose-containing foods – include cramps, wind, bloating, diarrhoea and sometimes nausea. It's a common condition, affecting about 5 per cent of the adult population. Many people become increasingly lactose intolerant as they get older.

If you have this problem, it doesn't necessarily prevent you from consuming yoghurt and other dairy products. Some tips:

• Try yoghurt, kefir or aged cheese. The probiotics they contain actually break down lactose. Consequently, many lactose-intolerant individuals are able to eat them. Similarly, you may find that aged cheese doesn't trigger symptoms.

• Spread out your dairy consumption. For example, if you experience gastrointestinal distress from a full pot of yoghurt, try four quarter-pot servings consumed several hours apart.

• Take a supplement containing the lactase enzyme (available at chemists and health food stores) as you begin to eat or drink a food with lactose. The enzyme breaks down the lactose and often prevents symptoms.

Even if you're too lactose intolerant for these measures to help, you can still get the benefits of probiotics from soya yoghurt and from the other fermented foods described in this chapter. Supplements are another option, which I'll discuss in Chapter 11.

Many foods that used to be prepared by fermentation, such as pickles, gherkins and sauerkraut, are now prepared by chemical treatment. Though this simplifies their manufacture and makes their shelf life longer, it means that these products are no longer a source of probiotics. However, you can still find traditional fermented foods, if you know where and how to look. Here are a few examples.

Pickles or gherkins

In our grandparents' time, almost all pickles were made by fermentation. Fresh cucumbers (or other vegetables or fruit) were placed in large vats of heavily salted water, called brine. This pulled the sugar from inside the cucumber to the surface, where lactic acid bacteria – already naturally present – could use it as food. Over several weeks, the pickles would ferment and become sour. Today, most gherkins sold in grocery stores are not fermented but simply soaked in vinegar. The vinegar preserves the cucumber and also changes its flavour and texture to that of a gherkin. But it doesn't add probiotic bacteria.

Naturally fermented gherkins – which contain probiotics – are still available. But you'll need to search for them and read the labels. Look for gherkins that are packed in brine and that don't contain vinegar as an ingredient. If they're packed in jars, you'll find them in the refrigerated section. I prefer these gherkins to the usual vinegary kind, not only for their probiotics but also for their nice fresh flavour.

Sauerkraut

Sauerkraut is German for 'sour cabbage'. Traditional sauerkraut is made by shredding cabbage, mixing it with salt and allowing it to ferment. Read the label to make sure that you're buying a naturally fermented version. As with gherkins, you'll find sauerkraut with live bacteria in the refrigerated section. Sauerkraut is low in calories and high in fibre. It provides both flavour and probiotics when consumed uncooked. In addition to using it as a condiment and in sandwiches, try adding it to salads and dips. Cooked sauerkraut doesn't contain live bacteria, but does retain its prebiotic and metabiotic content.

Kimchi

When *Health* magazine selected the five healthiest foods in the world, the shortlist included kimchi, a popular Korean condiment made from fermented cabbage and sometimes additional vegetables (such as radish, red pepper and onion), plus salt, garlic, chilli pepper, ginger and other spices. Look for kimchi in large supermarkets, Asian food stores and health food stores. As you might guess from the list of ingredients, kimchi can be dauntingly hot. But some versions are relatively mild. (By the way, yoghurt made the magazine's 'healthiest foods' list, too.)

➤ A NUTRITIONIST SPEAKS ABOUT KIMCHI ➤

Dana Reed, MS, CNS, CDN, is a nutritionist in private practice who also teaches at the Tri-State College of Acupuncture in New York City. She describes how she learnt about the benefits of kimchi:

Some years ago, before I became a nutritionist, I was in Korea on business. I had a long history of digestion problems and the combination of jet lag and going out to dinner set it off quite badly. I was up all night with stomach pains, running to the toilet. The next day, I wasn't looking very good. My Korean colleagues asked what the matter was. When I explained that I was having difficulty adjusting to the food, they said, 'We always have a little kimchi with it, to aid digestion.'

At the time, I didn't know how kimchi was made or why it would be beneficial – I found all that out afterwards. Because it's strong-tasting, I eased my way into it. There are many versions of kimchi, and my colleagues offered me different forms to try. Some weren't quite as spicy as others. I can't say that I loved it immediately, but it didn't take long to develop a taste for it. And it did help with my digestive issues in combination with other factors. I also became more careful about trying new foods. I'd take just a little bit and have kimchi with it. I'd avoid foods I learnt were 'triggers', and also incorporated other fermented foods into my diet.

Since then, I have done a fair amount of research on the health benefits of fermented foods. They are an integral part of my practice.

Miso

If you enjoy Japanese food, you're probably familiar with miso soup – but perhaps not with miso itself. Miso (pronounced 'MEE-so') is a paste made from soya beans, cultured grain and salt. It's blended and then fermented for months or even years. You can find miso at Asian supermarkets, as well as at many large supermarkets and health food stores. Try it as a seasoning, to replace all or part of the salt in recipes for soups, salads, pasta, stews and other dishes.

It's simpler to pop supplements than to make dietary changes. But I hope you'll add probiotic-rich foods to your diet. They undoubtedly contain beneficial substances we haven't yet discovered. And they also taste very good!

➤ SUPERMARKET WATCH ◀

Here are new products you can expect to see in the future – indeed, some are available now (though not always easily found in Britain yet). Time will tell if these are useful additions to the diet or merely marketing gimmicks.

• **Super cheeses:** Cheese is an excellent medium for culturing bacteria and keeping them alive. Probiotic-enriched super cheeses are already sold in Europe.

• **Probiotic-enriched fruit juices, teas and water:** These beverages are popular in Europe and Japan and are starting to also be available in Britain.

• **Snacks and breakfast cereals:** Someday, thanks to a new technology called microencapsulation, food manufacturers will be able to add live probiotic bacteria to dry foods like crisps, crackers and breakfast cereals, which are stored at room temperature. The bacteria – which normally could not survive under these conditions – will be surrounded with a temporary protective coating made from vegetable fatty acids or other edible ingredients. Only when the food is consumed and reaches the intestines will the coating dissolve, delivering probiotics to the gut.

Though microencapsulation is still under development, some cereals already include dried probiotics. Examples of this first wave of probiotic-enriched cereals are Kashi's Vive Probiotic Digestive Wellness Cereal and YogActive Cereal (not yet readily available in Britain). Currently, the labels don't tell us the types and numbers of probiotics contained, their shelf life or their viability at the time of the expiry date. I eagerly await more information from the manufacturers and from clinical research that uses these innovative foods.

- **Products for children:** Some yoghurts are sold in containers with kid appeal. Some manufacturers also offer kefir in flavours like orange and lime to appeal to children.

- **Foods with added prebiotics:** Now arriving in European shops arc beverages and foods enriched with *prebiotics*. Examples include flavoured water, bread, energy bars – and even a chocolate spread.

CHAPTER ELEVEN

Choosing Probiotic Supplements

Supplements were part of my plan when I decided to see if probiotics could address my allergies and asthma. I've always enjoyed yoghurt and cheese (and later discovered kefir as well). But I expected to need high doses of probiotics. I was concerned that if I attempted to get the full amount from food, my diet would become unbalanced.

Probiotic supplements are an important option for many people. If you're hoping to treat a specific illness, or trying to counter the side effects of antibiotic treatment, food sources may not be sufficient to get the job done – as was the case for me. Supplements can deliver the powerful therapeutic hit you need. Or you may wish to use particular patented microbes, some found only in supplements, that have been clinically tested either for overall health or for a medical problem that concerns you.

Taking supplements is a way to gain the benefits of probiotics when dietary changes are difficult. For example, if you're lactose intolerant or allergic to dairy products, it's not easy to get sufficient probiotics from food. The same is often true when you're travelling or if you eat most of your meals away from home.

Shopping for probiotic supplements can be confusing. The first time I went to my local health food store to buy a probiotic supplement, I was astonished – and overwhelmed – by the selection. I found numerous brands. Probiotics were sold as powders, capsules, pills and liquids. Some supplements were refrigerated; others were not. I spent nearly an hour reading labels before making my selection. Later, as I worked on this book, I spent even more time tracking down brands, scrutinising labels and reading research reports.

This chapter will help you sort through the options. I'll tell you what to look for and give you a quick checklist to take to the store. I'll also suggest how to work out an appropriate dose and explain how to use supplements to optimal advantage. Though I'll mention specific brands, I want you to know that as I prepared this information, I had no commercial connections to any products or retailers.

Even if you plan to take probiotic supplements, I hope you'll also make the dietary changes recommended in this book. Think of all the nutrients you get – vitamins, minerals, antioxidants and protein – along with the friendly microbes in probiotic-rich foods. In addition, food delivers probiotics to the lining of your mouth. If your only source is a capsule that takes the express route to your stomach, you're missing the added benefits of probiotics in fighting cavities and bad breath. And let's not forget that it's a lot more enjoyable to eat delicious food than to swallow a supplement, valuable as that supplement might be.

HOW PROBIOTIC SUPPLEMENTS ARE MADE

Microbes destined for supplements often originate in humans, so we know they're compatible with our body. They're grown in huge fermentation vessels, which are similar to those used to make beer. Once the microbes reach high concentrations, the liquid is drained off with a centrifuge. The microbes are rinsed several times with clean water or salt solutions – a process similar to rinsing and spinning clothing in a washing machine. Most of the microbes are used to make supplements. But some are saved to produce more. High-quality probiotic supplements list a batch or lot number on the bottle.

The best method for extending the life of a microbe is to remove the water from it. This is done by freeze-drying: the rinsed and drained microbes are frozen, and all the fluid is removed by vacuum. What remains is a powder that consists of dried probiotic microbes. This powder is packaged in various forms: in bottles, in individual capsules or packets, pressed into tablets or in liquids. When the supplements are taken, and the powder is exposed to fluid, the microbes return to life.

IMPORTANT CAUTIONS

All the probiotic strains used in the supplements discussed in this chapter are considered safe to consume, even at very high doses. This includes probiotics in the *Bifidobacterium* species, *Lactobacillus* species, *Streptococcus thermophilus* (used as a yoghurt starter), *Propionibacterium* (used as a cheese starter), *Lactococcus lactis* (used as a buttermilk starter) and the probiotic yeast *Saccharomyces boulardii*.

There are no dangerous strains – or even species – of *Bifido-bacterium* or *Lactobacillus*. However, a few supplements use probiotic

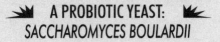

A PROBIOTIC YEAST: SACCHAROMYCES BOULARDII

Most of the microbes used for probiotic supplements are bacteria. However, one valuable probiotic is a yeast. It was discovered in the 1920s by Henri Boulard, a French microbiologist, during his travels in South-east Asia. While visiting a village hit by infectious diarrhoea, he observed that people successfully countered the symptoms by drinking an infusion made by boiling the skins of lychee fruit. Boulard was able to isolate the curative ingredient from this beverage, a yeast microbe. Since it was similar to the yeast used to make bread – *Saccharomyces cerevisiae* – he named it *Saccharomyces boulardii*. (Some scientists now believe that Boulard's discovery is really a close relative of *Saccharomyces cerevisiae*, which is why the same microbe is sometimes referred to as *Saccharomyces cerevisiae* ssp *boulardii*.)

A commercially developed strain of S. *boulardii*, *Saccharomyces boulardii* lyo – available in some kefirs and supplements – has been widely used by physicians in Europe for treating antibiotic-induced diarrhoea, adult and childhood acute diarrhoea and diarrhoea associated with *Clostridium difficile*. After years of clinical studies, two recent medical reports recommended its use by American physicians for these types of diarrhoea.

strains of other microbes that are very similar to strains that cause life-threatening disease. Some of these probiotic strains are developing an impressive clinical record for treating specific diseases. Nevertheless, because certain disease-causing and probiotic strains are similar, I recommend that you consult your healthcare practitioner before consuming supplements containing strains of *E. coli*, *Enterococcus faecium* or *Bacillus subtilis*.

Some especially vulnerable individuals can develop dangerous infections from probiotic microbes – even those that are generally considered safe. Though such problems are extremely rare, it's important to consult a healthcare practitioner before taking any probiotic supplement, whether yeast or bacteria, if you:

• have an immunodeficiency disease, such as AIDS
• are taking an immunosuppressive drug, such as ones used to treat autoimmune diseases or to prevent the rejection of transplanted organs
• are receiving chemotherapy or radiation therapy
• are under medical care for a serious digestive tract disorder
• have ever experienced an adverse reaction to a probiotic formulation
• are hospitalised for any reason

In addition to the cautions above, be sure to ask for professional medical guidance before taking the probiotic yeast *Saccharomyces boulardii* if you:

• are pregnant (and therefore more vulnerable to yeast infections)
• have ever suffered an adverse reaction to yeast or yeast products

Because *Saccharomyces boulardii* treats infectious diarrhoea so effectively, your physician may prescribe this probiotic even if you have one of the conditions above. Under such circumstances, you should be closely monitored for any unfavourable reactions.

➤ GUIDANCE FOR DOCTORS ➤

In 2005, a panel of doctors and other experts in the field of probiotics and digestive diseases held a workshop at the Yale University School of Medicine. Participants analysed the growing number of probiotics clinical trials and developed guidelines for clinicians based on this review. Their recommendations were published in the *Journal of Clinical Gastroenterology* in 2006.

According to the panel's guidelines, probiotics are recommended for treatment of acute diarrhoea, antibiotic-associated diarrhoea and ileal pouchitis (an infection discussed in the box on page 115). They also pointed to studies showing that probiotics can improve immune response. In addition, the panel noted accumulating evidence that probiotics may be of benefit in treating *Helicobacter pylori* infection, radiation-associated diarrhoea, vaginal infections, ulcerative colitis, Crohn's disease and irritable bowel syndrome.

The panel's published guidelines included citations to sixty-one scientific studies. They suggested that clinicians use the study protocols to determine the type of probiotic and dose to use with patients. The recommendations in this book include that advice.

HOW MUCH DO YOU NEED?

This question is the subject of ongoing research and intense debate. As I explained in Chapter 10, we don't yet have precise guidelines for optimal intake of probiotics, whether in food or in supplements. But everyone agrees that supplement dosing depends upon treatment goals. The more ambitious the goal, the higher the suggested daily dose – that is, the higher the number of live microbes.

Food labels usually refer to live bacteria or live cultures. Supplement labels usually describe the microbial contents as 'colony-forming units' (CFU), meaning the number of microbes – either bacteria or yeasts – that are capable of dividing and forming colonies. That's just a fancy way of saying 'live and healthy microbes'. The numbers, typically in the billions, may sound staggering. But one serving of yoghurt with live bacteria contains billions of microbes, too.

The following suggestions are based on typical doses given to patients in scientific studies that use supplements to prevent or treat disease. This indicates that they've been found both safe and effective in these amounts. Consider these numbers to be starting points. Each person is different; you may need a higher dose to get the desired results – or you may find that a smaller amount is sufficient. In Chapter 14, I'll explain how to make adjustments, depending on how your body responds.

To Maintain Good Health

If you're simply hoping to maintain good health, you can get all the probiotics you need from food; just follow the recommendations in Chapter 10. Should you prefer to take a supplement – for example, if you're lactose intolerant or if you'd like to use a particular strain available only in supplement form – begin with a dose of at least 3 to 5 billion CFU per day. That's comparable to what's been used in studies of healthy people to see if probiotics can ward off minor illnesses. For example, students in the academic stress study I described in Chapter 5 simply drank a probiotic shot.

To Improve Health or Prevent a Health Problem

Aim for 6 to 10 billion CFU per day if you have a specific health concern; consuming more is not a problem. For example, Dr Michael Cabana – who is leading the University of California, San Francisco, USA, asthma prevention study I described in Chapter 7 – is providing probiotics to half of the pregnant women participating in the investigation; the rest will receive a placebo. All of the babies are at elevated risk for asthma because one or both of their parents have the condition. Dr Cabana and his associates hope to learn if probiotics can reduce this risk. The mums-to-be who are given probiotics will receive 10 billion CFU per day.

Similar doses have been used in research throughout the life cycle. New Zealand investigators gave 30 healthy older volunteers – men and women aged 63 to 84 – daily supplements of 5 billion bacteria, which were consumed in milk. Over a three-week period, this amount increased their immune function, as measured by changes in their white blood cells. None of the participants experienced any unfavourable reactions to the supplements.

To Treat a Mild to Moderate Health Condition

Use 20 to 30 billion CFU per day to address a medical problem. Doses in this range have been proven effective in a wide variety of conditions. A few examples:

• Two doses of probiotics, totalling 24 billion CFU per day, were used in a Polish study of young children who were hospitalised with acute infectious diarrhoea. This amount significantly shortened the duration of their illness. Despite the fact that probiotics were administered to 87 vulnerable children aged 2 months to 6 years, no adverse side effects were seen.

• In a Danish investigation, atopic dermatitis was successfully treated in children aged 1 to 13 with a probiotic dose of 20 billion CFU per day. The children participated in the study for eighteen weeks. They were divided into two groups, each taking a placebo or supplement for six weeks, stopping for six weeks and then switching to the other treatment (supplement or placebo) for the final six weeks. During the placebo period, eczema symptoms improved in just 15 per cent of the patients – but while they were taking probiotics, 56 per cent saw improvements.

TRAVELLERS' DIARRHOEA

If you're using probiotics to prevent travellers' diarrhoea, here are some suggestions:

• Stack the odds in your favour by consuming lots of probiotics before you go – at least one serving of yoghurt or kefir per day or supplements supplying 10 billion CFU.

• Pack supplements when you travel, selecting ones with multiple strains. It's okay not to refrigerate them for one or two weeks. *Saccharomyces boulardii*, a probiotic yeast that's effective against diarrhoea, needs no refrigeration.

• Consume at least 10 billion CFU daily. If you're in a region where travellers' diarrhoea is a common problem, aim for a total of 20 to 30 billion CFU daily, taken in two or three doses spread throughout the day.

Don't neglect the usual advice to watch what you eat and drink:

• Use only sealed bottled water, or water that's been boiled, for drinking, making ice, washing fruit and vegetables and cleaning your teeth.

• Avoid unpasteurised dairy products, as well as raw or undercooked meat, poultry and seafood.

• Peel fruit and vegetables, even if you would normally eat the skins.

(See the box titled 'If You're Taking Antibiotics', on pages 242–243, for advice on when diarrhoea warrants a call to the doctor.)

• A team of Polish and Swedish scientists studied the effects of probiotics on cardiovascular risk factors in heavy smokers. For six weeks, half of them received a daily rose hip drink that contained 20 billion CFU; the others, the control group, were given the same drink without probiotic bacteria. At the end of six weeks, blood pressure was significantly lower in those in the probiotics group, but unchanged in the controls.

For my own treatment plan, I aimed for three servings per day of probiotic-rich foods. To treat my allergies and asthma, I added probiotic supplements that supplied another 6 to 10 billion bacteria daily. Once my allergies and asthma were under control, and I was simply trying to maintain good health, I cut my supplement intake in half. But I still consume two servings per day of yoghurt, cheese or kefir.

To Treat Severe Disease

If you have a serious medical problem, you should be under the care of a licensed healthcare practitioner. Probiotic treatment could involve high doses, given along with other medications. VSL#3 is a probiotic product that contains 450 billion CFU per packet, many times more than other supplements. In clinical studies, patients have been treated with multiple packets per day of VSL#3, doses that add up to a total daily bacteria count well in the trillions.

VSL#3 is available without a prescription. You can purchase it online or at some local chemists or health food stores; stores that don't carry it are sometimes willing to order it. However, it's marketed as a 'medical food' rather than as a nutritional supplement. The Food and Drug Administration defines medical foods as products prescribed by a physician to manage a specific medical condition. Like prescription drugs, medical foods are intended to be taken under professional supervision.

✺ IF YOU'RE TAKING ANTIBIOTICS ✺

Probiotics are a proven way to prevent and treat common side effects of antibiotics, especially diarrhoea. When you need to take an antibiotic, protect your microflora:

• If you know beforehand that you're beginning a course of antibiotics, take an extra dose of probiotics a few days beforehand. A dose in this case is a serving of yoghurt or kefir, or an additional supplement with at least 10 billion CFU.

• Once you begin the medication, take a total of two or more doses of probiotics during the day. But don't consume them with antibiotics. If they're in your stomach at the same time, the probiotics will be massacred. Keeping your gut supplied with probiotics is an uphill battle, because many will be killed by the antibiotics even if you take them separately. And if you already have diarrhoea when you start probiotics, many will be running through your digestive tract with no opportunity to colonise. Don't worry that the probiotics might interfere with the antibiotics: the drug can kill trillions of microbes, so even repeated 10 billion CFU doses of probiotics don't hold them back.

• Try to consume a wide variety of probiotics. Use multiple sources – say, yoghurt plus kefir or two supplements that contain different microbes – or look for a single source with at least six different probiotics. An exception: if your doctor advises you to avoid dairy products (for example, if a tetracycline-based antibiotic is prescribed) or if you find they disagree with you, supplements are best.

Consider including *Saccharomyces boulardii* (contained in many formulations of kefir and in Florastor) and *Lactobacillus rhamnosus* GG (Culturelle); both have been found effective against antibiotic-associated diarrhoea, though various probiotic blends also work. Because *Saccharomyces boulardii* is a yeast, it will be impervious to the antibiotic, even if they're taken together.

• Continue taking at least one extra dose of probiotics per day for at least a week after your course of antibiotics is finished. The battle in your GI tract doesn't end when you go off the medication.

• Throughout the process, try to eat well: keep prebiotics high (fruit, vegetables, whole grains) and refined carbohydrates (sugary foods) low. This gives probiotics a supportive environment and helps them to compete.

An important caveat: most of the time, antibiotic-associated diarrhoea is a temporary annoyance; the problem is resolved in a few days, even without treatment. Probiotics can help speed recovery. But do-it-yourself remedies are appropriate only for what Michigan State University infectious disease specialist Dr Vincent Young calls 'nuisance' diarrhoea. His advice: seek medical attention promptly if you develop any of the following symptoms in addition to diarrhoea; they could indicate a more serious problem:

• abdominal pain
• blood in the stool
• fever
• signs of dehydration, such as feeling dizzy when you stand up.

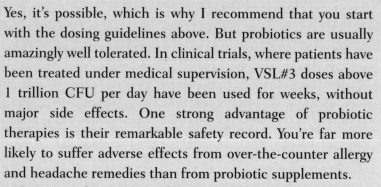

⋟ CAN PROBIOTIC SUPPLEMENTS CAUSE ⋞ ADVERSE SIDE EFFECTS?

Yes, it's possible, which is why I recommend that you start with the dosing guidelines above. But probiotics are usually amazingly well tolerated. In clinical trials, where patients have been treated under medical supervision, VSL#3 doses above 1 trillion CFU per day have been used for weeks, without major side effects. One strong advantage of probiotic therapies is their remarkable safety record. You're far more likely to suffer adverse effects from over-the-counter allergy and headache remedies than from probiotic supplements.

Some people experience flatulence, bloating or (more rarely) diarrhoea when they begin, especially if doses are high. The effect is similar to what sometimes occurs if a person suddenly increases their fibre intake. Fortunately, these difficulties aren't dangerous; they usually disappear on their own as your body adjusts. If you experience troublesome symptoms of this nature when you take supplements, simply reduce the dose. After the problems go away, gradually increase your intake until you reach the desired amount.

PROBIOTIC STRAINS TO TAKE

No matter what your goal, I recommend that you select foods and supplements that provide a variety of probiotic microbes. Be sure to include members of both the *Lactobacillus* and *Bifidobacterium* groups.

What if there's a particular strain that's been proven effective against a medical condition you're hoping to address? If so, the strain is definitely worth including in the mix – see the table at the end of this chapter for a list of strains for which there's evidence of therapeutic value. But go for variety, too. Your chances for success are much greater if you consume a variety of probiotics via food or supplements or both.

Remember that scientists usually investigate only one strain at a time. That way, they know exactly why a particular treatment was or was not effective. However, only a small fraction of available strains have been tested. For instance, *Lactobacillus rhamnosus* GG (trade name: *Lactobacillus* GG) is a patented probiotic bacterial strain that has been studied extensively. Few other strains in the *Lactobacillus rhamnosus* species have received this kind of scientific attention. But all members of the species share many microbiological and biochemical traits, and others might be just as beneficial as – or even superior to – the GG strain. I believe that many probiotic species and strains ultimately will be found to be effective against specific conditions. Until all the information is in, variety is your best bet.

WHERE TO BUY PROBIOTIC SUPPLEMENTS

These days, probiotic supplements are sold by many health food stores and chemists, but you're more likely to find a wide selection in shops that specialise in vitamins and other nutritional supplements. In addition, many supplements can be purchased online or by telephone, either directly from the manufacturer or from a distributor.

It's best to obtain supplements from a source where they're kept under refrigeration. Also consider if the store is likely to sell these products regularly and replenish its stock frequently. Unlike vitamin pills, probiotic supplements contain living organisms. Though the microbes are in a powdered form that extends their lives, if they're not properly stored – or if they're stored too long – they can die even before you buy them. Keeping supplements cold slows their metabolism, almost putting them into a state of suspended animation.

This advice doesn't rule out mail-order sources, but it does mean you should plan ahead. Probiotics can survive several days without refrigeration, provided that they don't encounter hot weather (i.e., temperatures above 27°C) during transit. If you rely on mail order, stock up before summer.

One supplement that doesn't require refrigeration is Florastor, which contains the probiotic yeast *Saccharomyces boulardii* lyo. Though testing has shown that the yeast can survive at room temperature, I recommend refrigerating Florastor anyway, especially during hot weather. Refrigeration can't hurt, and it serves as insurance against unexpectedly high temperatures.

Scientists are developing new ways to keep probiotics alive longer without refrigeration. Chapter 10 mentioned one such technique, microencapsulation, which is already used in some food products. This method encapsulates probiotic microbes with a dissolvable coating that prevents them from dying at room temperature.

WHAT TO LOOK FOR

Shopping for a probiotic supplement can seem exceedingly complicated at first. But it's a lot easier if you know how to narrow down the abundant choices. Here are step-by-step suggestions.

Select a Reputable Brand

I have nothing against generics or store brands; I often select them when I'm buying an over-the-counter medication, such as a painkiller or decongestant. But probiotics and other dietary supplements aren't regulated the way drugs are. The Food and

Drug Administration (FDA) in the United States can step in if a supplement is found to be hazardous, but neither the FDA nor any other government agency tests or analyses them before they reach consumers. There's no guarantee that products actually contain the strains listed on the label, or that the microbes are still viable when you buy them – or that they're free from contamination. Responsibility for quality control is left to the manufacturer. In this 'buyer beware' market, I want to know who makes the probiotics I use.

The short list of supplement brands in the following table is not comprehensive; it includes those I've used myself or would give to my own family. Also included are the probiotic 'shots' I described in Chapter 10. These brands contain probiotic strains that have been used in peer-reviewed scientific studies with human subjects; the companies have good reputations for offering probiotics products that contain the expected number of live microbes.

While it's possible that a generic or store brand supplement could contain potentially pathogenic microbes, ineffective products are far more common than unsafe ones. ConsumerLab, a respected independent testing service, found in a 2003 study of 25 probiotic products that about a third of them contained less than 1 per cent of the expected number of live bacteria. In 2006, the situation was even worse. Only 8 of 13 probiotic supplements passed ConsumerLab's tests. Four of the products that failed provided fewer than 1 billion organisms, the minimum amount considered useful; the fifth met the minimum, but didn't contain the number of bacteria claimed. Similarly, when *Consumer Reports* tested 18 probiotic supplements in 2005, 7 of them contained far fewer living microbes than the label promised. However, none of the products involved in these tests was contaminated by harmful bacteria, moulds or fungi. Studies performed elsewhere have reached similar conclusions.

RECOMMENDED BRANDS OF PROBIOTIC SUPPLEMENTS AND SHOTS

(For purchasing information, see websites or ring. Some supplements are available at chemists or health food stores. Shots are sold in supermarkets and health food stores.)

SUPPLEMENT BRAND	CONTAINS
Culturelle http://www.culturelle.com (USA only) 001-888-828-4242	10 billion CFU per capsule *Lactobacillus rhamnosus* GG (trade name *Lactobacillus* GG)
Florastor http://www.florastor.com	5 billion CFU per capsule *Saccharomyces boulardii* lyo (a probiotic yeast)
Jarrow-dophilus Jarrow http://www.jarrow.com (USA only) 001-800-726-0886	3.4 billion CFU per capsule *Lactobacillus rhamnosus* R0011, *L. casei* R0215, *L. acidophilus* R0052, *L. plantarum* R1012, *Bifidobacterium longum* BB536 (Morinaga), *B. breve* R0070
Fem-dophilus Jarrow http://www.jarrow.com (USA only) 001-800-726-0886	5 billion CFU per capsule *Lactobacillus rhamnosus* GR-1, *L. reuteri* RC-14
Theralac http://www.theralac.com (USA only) 001-800-926-2961	20 billion CFU per capsule *Lactobacillus rhamnosus* HN001, *L. paracasei* F-19, *L. acidophilus*, *Bifidobacterium lactis* HN019, *B. bifidum* BB-12
VSL#3 http://www.vsl3.com (USA only) 001-866-438-8753 Note: VSL#3 is a medical food, to be taken under a doctor's supervision.	450 billion CFU per packet *Bifidobacterium breve, B. longum, B. infantis, Lactobacillus acidophilus, L. plantarum, L. casei, L. bulgaricus, Streptococcus thermophilus*

SHOT BRAND	CONTAINS
Activia http://www.danoneactivia.co.uk	10 billion bacteria per 120 ml container *Lactobacillus bulgaricus, Streptococcus thermophilus, Bifidobacterium animalis* DN-173 010 (trade name: *Bifidus Regularis*)
Actimel http://www.uk.actimel.com	10 billion bacteria per 100 ml bottle *Lactobacillus casei* DN-114 001 (trade name *L. casei* Defensis or *L. casei* Immunitas), *L. bulgaricus, Streptococcus thermophilus*
Yakult http://www.yakult.co.jp/english	6.5 billion bacteria per 70 ml bottle *Lactobacillus casei* Shirota

I want to emphasise that this list is not complete. Because I'm a scientist, I've focused on brands that have been used in research. Your healthcare adviser may have different suggestions, based on years of experience with patients. Here are other ways to find reliable brands:

• Check the reports of ConsumerLab (http://www.consumerlab.com) or other consumer organisations that test probiotic supplements to learn whether a brand contains the listed number of viable microbes. ConsumerLab has a voluntary testing programme for manufacturers. Products that pass their tests are listed on their website and are permitted to carry the CL certification seal.
• Select supplements from companies that also produce drugs or food, since they're held to strict standards for those products.
• Check the manufacturer's website to assess their commitment to quality and to see if they're following good manufacturing processes. Favourable signs include: citations to scientific studies

published in peer-reviewed journals that use their products or strains contained in their products; evidence that they've set standards and can document that they follow these standards (for example, they submit their products to independent laboratories for testing).

Choose Products That List Probiotics by Genus, Species and Strain

Check the supplement's label to see what microbes are included. Choose supplements that list the particular genus, species and strain of the probiotics contained – for example, not merely *Bifidobacterium* or *Bifidobacterium lactis*, but *Bifidobacterium lactis* HN019. That's a promising sign of quality control. Avoid supplements that simply use the term 'proprietary blend' instead of providing a list.

Full information is especially important if you're hoping to reap the benefits of a particular strain. Each genus contains many species. One example: scientists have identified dozens of species of *Lactobacillus,* including *L. rhamnosus, L. casei, L. acidophilus* and many others. Within these species are numerous strains. Not all of the strains have the same effects in the body. For instance, *Lactobacillus rhamnosus* GG has been shown to reduce the side effects of triple therapy for ulcers. However, we can't assume that other species of *Lactobacillus* – or even other strains of *Lactobacillus rhamnosus* – provide the same benefit. The table at the end of the chapter includes the probiotic strains found most effective in scientific studies.

➤➤ RESEARCHING THE SCIENTIFIC LITERATURE ➤➤

Has a particular probiotic strain been clinically tested? Is there any new scientific research on treating a particular disease with probiotics? Thanks to the Internet, it's easy to find out.

Peer-reviewed scientific studies – ones that are checked by other scientists before publication – are indexed by the National Library of Medicine (NLM). Together with the National Institutes of Health, NLM also provides a free service called PubMed (http://www.pubmed.com) that allows you to search the index. Simply type in a search term, such as the name of a probiotic strain or a disease, and press 'Enter' on your keyboard. PubMed will search over 13 million reports from more than 4,800 scientific journals and present you with a list of citations to relevant studies. Use the pull-down 'Display' menu near the top of that screen to select 'Abstract' if you would like to see a summary of each study.

In most cases, you can read a study abstract (a brief summary) online at no charge – at least if the study was published in the past few years. For recent studies, the full text is likely to be available as well; however, there may be a hefty charge to read it. Sometimes you can find complete medical journal articles online via an Internet search engine. Google Scholar (http://scholar.google.com) can be particularly useful.

Look for Microbe Counts

Most supplement manufacturers clearly state the number of CFUs – colony-forming units (live microbes) – contained in their supplements. You need this information to determine how much to take; it will also help you compare prices (see the box on the next page).

Be wary of manufacturers that give you the weight of their products in grams, milligrams or millilitres instead of providing microbe counts. Unfortunately, the weight tells you nothing about the microbial contents. How much a capsule or packet weighs depends not only on the number of probiotic organisms it contains, but also upon how the supplement was manufactured and what other ingredients it includes. For example, extra salt could add to the weight – but not to the probiotic value of a supplement.

Select Capsules or Single-Use Packets

The best method for extending the life of a microbe is to remove the water from it, turning it into a powder. This would kill many living creatures, but it merely suspends the metabolic activity of a microbe. Restoring the water brings the microbe back to life.

The enemies of dried probiotic microbes are high temperature, water (unless added just prior to consumption) and air. In the future, microencapsulated probiotic strains will not need to be protected from the air, because microencapsulation will do just that. However, until the technology advances, I recommend supplements that are sealed in capsules or single-use packets.

Check the Expiry Date

Even with optimal storage, bacteria can't survive indefinitely. That's why the expiry date is important. Before you buy, work out if you can use up the supply before that date.

Consider the Extra Ingredients

Some probiotic supplements contain additional ingredients, such as prebiotics, herbs, vitamins or minerals. Another extra: enteric coatings. I give these additions mixed reviews.

➤ COMPARING PRICES ➤

When you shop for probiotics, you'll find that prices vary considerably. In general, brand name products with quality assurances cost more. Also, you usually pay more for capsules or packets that contain more CFU. That makes price comparisons tricky: a seemingly inexpensive product, with a low price per capsule, may be no bargain once you calculate the cost of a daily dose.

When I'm comparison shopping, I do a quick mental calculation to translate the price of each product into the cost per 5 billion CFU.

Cost-saving dos and don'ts:

Do –

☑ Compare prices from different vendors – including online sources. Be sure to include any charges for shipping.

☑ Open high-dose capsules or packets and split the dose between two days or two family members. Refrigerate any leftovers and use within a couple of days.

Don't –

☒ Buy in bulk if you can't finish the supply before the expiry date.

☒ Buy generic or store brands. There's a real risk of getting an inferior product that doesn't contain enough probiotics to achieve the results you're hoping for.

Does a Supplement Need a Supplement?

Adding prebiotics – such as inulin or FOS (fructo-oligosaccharide) – could be beneficial, since they help probiotic microbes to survive in the digestive tract. However, I'm less enthusiastic about supplements that contain herbs, vitamins, minerals or other ingredients beyond probiotic microbes and prebiotics.

My reasoning is the same for probiotic supplements as it is for cold medicines. I can buy a multi-ingredient cold medicine that takes care of aches, congestion, runny nose and coughing. But what if my cold doesn't involve aches or coughing? I don't want to take medications that I don't need. Therefore, I buy each component separately, and take only what's required to address my particular symptoms. Similarly, I prefer to buy probiotic and other supplements individually. Some herbs, vitamins and minerals can interact with medications; some can be harmful in high doses.

If you want to use an herbal supplement, buy it separately. This will give you more control over your total supplement intake.

Enteric Coatings

Enteric coatings allow medications to pass through the acidic environment of the stomach, so they can be released in the small intestine. However, effective probiotics can survive passage through the stomach without enteric coatings. Moreover, such a coating may restrict the product's usefulness for general health. For example, probiotics may be effective in reducing bad breath, gum disease and cavities – but not if they bypass the mouth. Similarly, they can help prevent stomach ulcers – provided that they reach the stomach.

Nevertheless, an enteric coating could be valuable under certain circumstances. Since the coating maximises the number of probiotic microbes that reach the intestinal tract, it might increase the effectiveness of a clinically proven probiotic strain if you're treating an intestinal condition, such as diarrhoea.

Ignore Meaningless Claims

Supplement packages or advertising may contain the following claims, none of which means a superior product.

'Clinically Effective'

Though some probiotic supplement labels legitimately say that the product is clinically effective, a much larger number of supplements make unsubstantiated claims of this nature. How can you tell the difference? Check the table at the end of the chapter to see if the strains contained in the supplement are listed. Go to the manufacturer's website and look for citations to studies. Or do your own research (see the box on page 251 about researching the scientific literature).

One common version of this claim is a statement like this one: 'Lactobacillus casei has been clinically proven to be effective at reducing antibiotic-associated diarrhoea.' The problem is that there are many strains of Lactobacillus casei. For example, L. casei DN-114 001 is indeed effective against diarrhoea associated with antibiotics. However, many other L. casei strains haven't yet been tested – and some may have been tested and found not to work.

'Guaranteed Analysis'

At the moment, there's no national standard or testing for probiotic supplements, so the promise of 'guaranteed analysis' – by itself – is meaningless. However, some supplement manufacturers do seek independent testing. How can you tell the difference? Look for the name of the laboratory that performed the tests, and expect the results to be readily available to any consumer who wants to check them. (See, for example, the quality assurance offered by Theralac at http://www.theralac.com.) This kind of specific information offers reassurance that the product is not contaminated and that it contains viable probiotics of the promised strains.

'Age-Specific Blend'

There's no data to support the claim that people of a particular age need a customised blend of probiotics. On the contrary, research suggests that people of all ages benefit in similar ways from particular strains. Focus on your health goals, not your age.

Similarly, men and women benefit from the same organisms. However, if you're a woman and one of your goals is to treat or prevent vaginal yeast infections, you might be particularly interested in the probiotics that have been found to colonise the vagina – see Chapter 8, page 162. At least one blend marketed to women, Jarrow's Fem-dophilus (see the list of supplements on page 248), contains such bacteria.

'Contains Supernatant' or 'Not Centrifuged'

To produce supplements, probiotic microbes are grown in a nutrient broth, which is called the supernatant. Before extracting water from the microbes themselves, the supernatant is removed by centrifugation. Some probiotics manufacturers say that adding supernatant to their products makes them more effective. Among the specific claims: 'Centrifuging damages the bacteria', 'The supernatant provides bacteria with nutrition during transportation and shelf storage time' and 'The supernatant protects bacteria from stomach acid.'

There's no scientific basis for these claims. The manufacturing process that leaves the probiotics dry and ready for packaging also removes or destroys most of the nutrients in the supernatant. So it wouldn't be possible to provide enough supernatant to nourish the bacteria. In any case, freeze-dried bacteria aren't metabolically active and don't require nutrition. Moreover, there's nothing in the supernatant that would protect bacteria from stomach acid. We know from laboratory analyses of properly stored probiotic supplements that bacteria survive the conventional manufacturing process – including centrifuging. And scientific studies show that they pass through the stomach in numbers large enough for the desired therapeutic effects.

GETTING THE MOST FROM SUPPLEMENTS

You can optimise the effectiveness of probiotic supplements by following these simple suggestions:

Consume with Food or Drink

Probiotic capsules can be effective if swallowed with a glass of water. However, I think the best way to take a supplement is to open the capsule or packet and either stir the contents into a beverage (e.g. milk, juice or water) or sprinkle them onto food (e.g. custard, yoghurt, jam). The powder has almost no flavour. To avoid killing the microbes, it's important for the food or drink to be no warmer than body temperature.

Consuming probiotics this way distributes them all along your gastrointestinal tract, starting with your mouth. Probiotic microbes may even migrate into the sinuses, where they can counter the harmful bacteria that cause sinus infections. In contrast, a capsule doesn't release its contents until it reaches the stomach. If you prefer to take a capsule, drink at least 120 ml of cool fluid with it. This helps rehydrate the freeze-dried microbes when the capsule dissolves inside your body.

Pair with Calcium

The best food or beverage to consume along with a probiotic supplement is one that contains calcium, such as yoghurt, milk or cheese. Calcium helps probiotic bacteria to adhere to the intestinal wall, while discouraging the adherence of harmful bacteria.

![] NEW WAYS TO DELIVER PROBIOTICS ![]

Here are some of the possibilities – most available now, others on the horizon.

• **Vaginal suppositories or douches:** Probiotics taken by mouth have been proven effective against vaginal yeast infections. What about delivering the same anti-yeast microbes directly, via suppository or douche? The idea is promising and such products are already on the market. However, they haven't yet been studied well enough for me to recommend them.

• **Anal suppositories:** Attempting to get probiotics into the intestines via suppositories means that you're fighting gravity and peristalsis. Anal suppositories are sold. But unless probiotic treatment is aimed at the low end of the colon, I'd be surprised if they worked well.

• **Powder applied to the skin:** Yeast infections are a common cause of nappy rash. On the horizon are probiotic powders that could be sprinkled on a baby's bottom to prevent rashes caused by yeast. So far, their effectiveness hasn't been well studied. Nor do we know if such powders – which could be inhaled by the baby – might cause allergic reactions.

• **Lozenges and chewing gum:** Probiotic lozenges and chewing gum are promising ways to counter bacteria in the mouth that cause tooth decay, bad breath and gum disease. Though their effectiveness hasn't yet been fully tested, probiotic lozenges are already available in the United States and a chewing gum supplement is being test-marketed in Sweden.

- **Probiotic-coated drinking straws and bottle caps:** Probiotic drinking straws and bottle caps are already marketed in Europe. The straws, designed for a single use, are coated on the inside with probiotic powder. As a beverage is sipped, the coating dissolves and is consumed along with the drink. The bottle caps hold a dose of probiotic powder, keeping it separate from the liquid. When it's time for a drink, the bottle is shaken and the powder blends with the fluid.

  These two inventions are clever and convenient. But they'll add to the cost of probiotic supplements. In the meantime, you can simply open a capsule, add it to the cold beverage of your choice and shake or stir.

- **Infant formula:** Baby formulas are among the foods that manufacturers are enriching with probiotics. Some products are already sold in Britain, and you can expect to see them in the supermarket soon. I look forward to studies of their effectiveness. (See page 281 for additional information about infant formulas.)

- **Other foods:** Probiotic 'shots', such as Actimel and Yakult, have already arrived; see the table on pages 248–249. And as I described in Chapter 10, manufacturers are marketing new foods – everything from breakfast cereal to chocolate spread – that contain added probiotics and prebiotics. Though there's good research to support the probiotic shots on my recommended list, I'm waiting for evidence about the rest.

If you are lactose intolerant, select non-dairy sources of calcium, like calcium-fortified orange juice or soya milk. But avoid products that contain calcium carbonate. These include not only some calcium supplements (check the label), but also many chewable antacids. While calcium carbonate is a good source of calcium, stomach acidity is actually helpful when you're taking probiotics: the acid kills most other bacteria, giving probiotic bacteria a competitive advantage not only in the stomach but also in the first part of the small intestine.

Split the Dose

If you're taking more than one supplement, divide your daily dose. Take half in the morning and the rest in the evening. This ensures that the intestinal tract is constantly seeded with probiotics, helping them to gain a competitive advantage over other microbes.

Store Properly

Keep probiotic supplements refrigerated and sealed in their capsules or packets. High temperature or exposure to air decreases their viability.

What if you're travelling, or if you need to take supplements when you're not at home? Fortunately, it's not necessary to pack them in ice. Most of the microbes will survive if they're kept at room temperature – but no higher – for a week or two. Just be sure not to leave them in a hot car. And don't get them wet. Rehydration brings the microbes out of suspended animation. At that point, they need to eat to survive. But since there's no food in a capsule or powder packet, they'll quickly die.

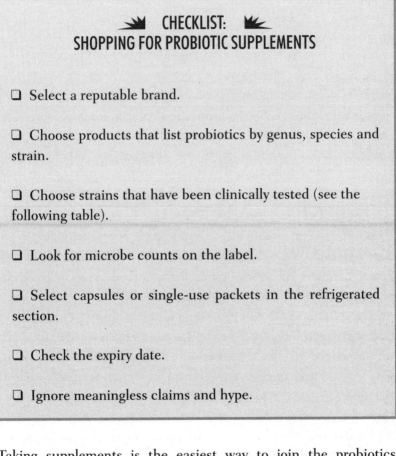

Use Promptly

It's tempting to purchase probiotic supplements in quantity to save money. But they'll be more potent if they're fresh.

➤ CHECKLIST: ◄
SHOPPING FOR PROBIOTIC SUPPLEMENTS

❑ Select a reputable brand.

❑ Choose products that list probiotics by genus, species and strain.

❑ Choose strains that have been clinically tested (see the following table).

❑ Look for microbe counts on the label.

❑ Select capsules or single-use packets in the refrigerated section.

❑ Check the expiry date.

❑ Ignore meaningless claims and hype.

Taking supplements is the easiest way to join the probiotics revolution. No dietary changes are required; even the busiest lifestyle is no obstacle. If you're unable to consume the probiotic-rich foods recommended in Chapter 10 – or if they simply don't appeal to you – consider trying a probiotic supplement.

The products described in this chapter have potential beyond their role as nutritional supplements. In capsules or powdered form, probiotics can be consumed in therapeutic doses that are much higher than would be feasible via fermented foods. As scientists and doctors explore the possibilities, we're beginning to discover that these friendly microbes provide a powerful yet safe way to treat many diseases.

A SUMMARY OF CURRENT RESEARCH

The following table summarises research findings to date on the health benefits of different probiotic strains and a few blends. All the probiotics listed have been investigated by scientists who published their results in peer-reviewed scientific journals. However, some have been studied more frequently or for more medical conditions than others.

I've divided the strains and blends into three general categories, depending on the amount of information currently available about them. In addition, I've indicated if particular probiotics have produced a positive response for various medical problems – or for overall good health and gastrointestinal health – in clinical (human) or research (animal) studies. The table highlights a few cases in which research findings are so favourable that a strain or blend was recommended by the 2005 Yale University workshop described on page 237, which developed guidelines for clinicians. Blank areas in the table mean either that studies had not yet been performed at the time this book went to press or that any investigations were inconclusive.

The table doesn't compare the quality of probiotic strains or supplement brands. Also, I want to emphasise that probiotics research is a very active field. Nearly every day, more studies are published and more results are reported. If you're curious about a particular strain or supplement, I encourage you to check PubMed,

CURRENT RESEARCH ON HEALTH BENEFITS OF PROBIOTIC STRAINS AND BLENDS

★: Strain or blend is recommended by the 2005 Yale University workshop (see page 237)

+: Strain has shown a positive response in human or animal studies

Genus	Species	Strain	General Health	GI Health	Inflammatory Bowel Disease	Irritable Bowel Syndrome	Viral Diarrhoea	Antibiotic-assoc Diarrhoea	C. difficile Diarrhoea	Travellers' Diarrhoea	Vaginal Yeast	Urinary Tract Infection	Eczema	Colds & Resp Virus	Allergy	Autoimmunity
Category 1: Significant number of clinical and research studies																
Bifidobacterium	animalis	DN-173 010, (1)	+	+												
Bifidobacterium	lactis	Bb-12	+	+			+						+			
Bifidobacterium	lactis	HN019, DR10	+	+			+									
Lactobacillus	acidophilus	NCFM	+	+		+	+									
Lactobacillus	casei	DN-114 001, (2)	+	+			+									
Lactobacillus	casei	Shirota	+	+	+			+							+	+
Lactobacillus	fermentum	RC-14	+	+							+	+				
Lactobacillus	plantarum	299v	+	+	+	+										
Lactobacillus	reuteri	SD2112, ING1, MM53, ATCC 55730, (3)	+	+			+			+				+		
Lactobacillus	rhamnosus	GG, LGG, (4)	+	+	+	+	★	★	+	+			+	+		
Lactobacillus	rhamnosus	GR-1	+	+							+	+				
Lactobacillus	rhamnosus	HN001, DR20	+	+		+									+	+
Saccharomyces	boulardii	lyo	+	+			★	★	★	+						
VSL#3, a blend of lactic acid bacteria (5)					★	★										

Category 2: Very promising clinical and research studies

Genus	Species	Strain	General Health	GI Health	Inflammatory Bowel Disease	Irritable Bowel Syndrome	Viral Diarrhoea	Antibiotic-assoc Diarrhoea	C. difficile Diarrhoea	Travellers' Diarrhoea	Vaginal Yeast	Urinary Tract Infection	Eczema	Colds & Resp Virus	Allergy	Autoimmunity
Bifidobacterium	breve	BR03, BR 03	+													
Bifidobacterium	breve	C50	+				+									
Bifidobacterium	breve	Yakult, BBG	+													
Bifidobacterium	breve	YIT4064	+				+									
Bifidobacterium	infantis	35624	+	+	+	+										
Bifidobacterium	longum	BB536, BB356	+	+											+	
Lactobacillus	acidophilus	DDS-1	+	+												
Lactobacillus	acidophilus	LA02, LA 02	+			+										
Lactobacillus	acidophilus	R0052, Rosell-52	+	+												
Lactobacillus	acidophilus	T20	+	+												
Lactobacillus	fermentum	B-54	+	+												
Lactobacillus	johnsonii	La1, NCC533, (6)	+	+												
Lactobacillus	paracasei	F19, (7)	+					+								
Lactobacillus	plantarum	LP01, LP 01	+			+										
Lactobacillus	reuteri	DSM 122460	+				+									
Lactobacillus	rhamnosus	19070-2	+				+						+			
Lactobacillus	rhamnosus	R0011, Rosell-11	+	+							+	+	+			
Lactobacillus	salivarius	UCC118	+	+	+											
Lactobacillus	salivarius	433118	+		+											

Category 3: Some published studies, either clinical or research

Genus	Species	Strain	General Health	GI Health	Inflammatory Bowel Disease	Irritable Bowel Syndrome	Viral Diarrhoea	Antibiotic-assoc Diarrhoea	C. difficile Diarrhoea	Travellers' Diarrhoea	Vaginal Yeast	Urinary Tract Infection	Eczema	Colds & Resp Virus	Allergy	Autoimmunity
Bifidobacterium	breve	BB99														
Bifidobacterium	longum	SBT-2928														
Lactobacillus	acidophilus	1748, NCFB 1748														
Lactobacillus	acidophilus	LA-1, LA-5														
Lactobacillus	acidophilus	SBT-2062														
Lactobacillus	crispatus	CTV05														
Lactobacillus	paracasei	33, LP33														
Lactobacillus	paracasei	CRL 431														
Lactobacillus	paracasei	ST11														
Lactobacillus	reuteri	CRL 1098														
Lactobacillus	rhamnosus	271														
Lactobacillus	rhamnosus	573L/1; 573L/2; 573L/3 (8)														

Probiotics and their trade names.

(1) *Bifidobacterium animalis* DN-173 010: Bifidus Regularis

(2) *Lactobacillus casei* DN-114 001: *L. casei* Defensis or *L. casei* Immunitas

(3) *Lactobacillus reuteri* SD2112 / 55730: *L. reuteri* Protectus, Reuteri ™

(4) *Lactobacillus rhamnosus* GG: *Lactobacillus* GG or LGG

(5) VSL# 3 is a probiotic blend containing strains of *Bifidobacterium breve, Bifidobacterium longum, Bifidobacterium infantis, Lactobacillus acidophilus, Lactobacillus plantarum, Lactobacillus casei, Lactobacillus bulgaricus* and *Streptococcus thermophilus* that are currently not identified by the manufacturer. Please refer to page 241 for more information about its status as a 'medical food'.

(6) *Lactobacillus johnsonii* La1: NCC533 or LC1

(7) *Lactobacillus paracasei* F19: *Lactobacillus* F19

(8) The mixture of *Lactobacillus rhamnosus* 573L/1, 573L/2 and 573L/3 is marketed as Lakcid L

as described in the box 'Researching the Scientific Literature' on page 251.

How can you find a supplement that contains a particular strain? Start by checking the list of recommended supplements on pages 248 to 249. Next, try searching online for the genus, species and strain name with Google or another Internet search engine. (A tip: put the entire name – genus, species, strain – in quotation marks, so the search results include only that particular strain.) Not all of the strains listed in the table are currently available commercially in Britain.

CHAPTER TWELVE

Prebiotics: Superstar Foods That Support Probiotics

With Mairi Noverr, PhD

Every time we eat, even if it's just a snack, we tinker with our microbial balance. Depending on the foods we select, we provide certain microbes with nutrients while making others go hungry. This chapter is about playing favourites – using prebiotics to create a congenial internal environment for friendly bacteria.

Prebiotics offer a cornucopia of healthy, delectable options. The chief sources are fruit, vegetables and whole grains. Prebiotics also are found in certain fats, tea, herbs and spices, red wine and – how's this for good news? – dark chocolate.

Dietary fibre is the best-known prebiotic. Our body can't digest fibre and turn it into fuel. But probiotic microbes thrive on it. Standard definitions of the term 'prebiotic' focus just on fibre. We think this definition needs to be expanded. Scientists now understand that fibre isn't the only food component that supports probiotics. I'll give you the expanded list, based on up-to-the-minute research that Mairi Noverr and I have assembled. You'll recognise some of these nutrients, because they're already known to have other important health benefits. When you nurture the beneficial microbes you host, you help your own body, too.

Prebiotics work in a variety of ways. Some feed probiotics; others slow down the microbes they compete against for survival. Also, some food compounds act like selective antibiotics, inhibiting the growth of particular microbes. Adding prebiotic-rich foods to your diet doesn't mean making drastic changes, especially if you're already following established guidelines for good nutrition or healthy weight loss. But you may find yourself looking at familiar foods in a whole new way – or even preparing them slightly differently.

FIBRE

Fibre is a form of carbohydrate, just like sugar and starch. But the human body doesn't produce enzymes that can break it down. When we consume foods containing fibre, the fibre passes right through our digestive tract. It provides us with no calories, vitamins or minerals. However, that doesn't mean it's useless. Along the way, fibre performs extremely valuable functions. One of the most important is that it serves as a prebiotic, selectively supporting probiotic microbes in our gut.

➤ CARBOHYDRATES 101 ➤

Carbohydrates are one of the three main nutrients in our diet, along with fats and proteins. The three most common carbohydrates are:

- Sugars, found mostly in fruit and vegetables

- Starches, primarily from grains and legumes

- Fibre, found in all foods of plant origin: grains, nuts, seeds, fruit and vegetables

When we digest sugars and starches, they're broken down into glucose, a simple form of sugar that's the body's chief energy source. Glucose enters the bloodstream, which delivers it to our cells. Fibre, which has no calories, isn't an energy source. But it helps our body to function in other important ways.

Types of Fibre

Fibre takes many different forms, but all of them can be grouped into two general categories – insoluble and soluble – depending on what happens when they're mixed with water. Insoluble fibre acts like a sponge: it holds water but doesn't dissolve. Soluble fibre behaves like a powder, absorbing water and forming a gel. Most plant foods contain both kinds of fibre, though one or the other may predominate – and both types are important for health. However, only soluble fibre acts as a prebiotic.

Insoluble Fibre

Insoluble fibre is sometimes called roughage, because it's coarse and bulky – characteristics that make important contributions to digestion and to good health. The bulk of insoluble fibre stimulates the intestines, helping food to move through them. This prevents not only constipation, but also conditions caused by straining and pressure in the colon, such as haemorrhoids and diverticulosis (a disorder in which infection-prone pouches form on the intestinal wall).

Some experts believe that insoluble fibre helps to prevent colon cancer: it picks up carcinogens and other toxins in our digestive tract, so they're not absorbed. In addition, insoluble fibre stimulates peristalsis, passing wastes out of the body more quickly. That means there's less opportunity for carcinogens to damage the intestinal lining. Think of insoluble fibre as a kind of disposable mop: it picks up potentially harmful substances and sweeps them away.

Insoluble fibre serves as a weight loss aid, too. The more such fibre a food contains, the bulkier it is and the more it contributes to a sense of fullness – yet insoluble fibre adds no calories. Fibre is the reason that most people find a piece of fruit more filling than a glass of juice.

Soluble Fibre

When soluble fibre absorbs water, it forms a sticky gel. This turns out to be useful for appetite control. When you eat something that contains both sugar and soluble fibre – say, an apple – its soluble fibre slows the release of its sugar. Take away the fibre, as with clear apple juice, and sugar enters the blood more rapidly. Both types of fibre offer bulk that lets you satisfy your appetite with fewer calories. And thanks to the soluble fibre, you stay satisfied for longer.

Soluble fibre also helps lower blood cholesterol levels. We don't know exactly how this works, but one explanation is that the sticky gel absorbs cholesterol and bile acids in the intestines. Bile acids are essential for digesting fats; they're made from cholesterol by the liver. Normally, any excess is reabsorbed by the body and recycled. But when bile acids are absorbed by soluble fibre, they get removed from the body as wastes. This forces the liver to produce more, which uses up cholesterol.

There's another mechanism that might explain the cholesterol-lowering benefit of soluble fibre: its role as a prebiotic. As I explained in Chapter 9, probiotics lower blood cholesterol levels – and soluble fibre favours the growth of probiotics.

➤ PREBIOTIC SUPER-FIBRES ◀

Two types of soluble fibre – oligosaccharides and inulin – are particularly helpful to probiotic bacteria. You may recognise their names from Chapters 10 and 11, because they're sometimes added to yoghurt and probiotic supplements. Increasingly, both of these fibres are being added to other prepared foods to boost their fibre content and to provide other health benefits. By the way, a food or supplement that contains both probiotics and prebiotics is sometimes called a 'synbiotic'.

• Oligosaccharides are a form of soluble fibre found in vegetables. We can't digest them, but probiotic microbes can. One oligosaccharide, fructo-oligosaccharide (FOS), is a particularly effective prebiotic. And a form of FOS called short-chain fructo-oligosaccharide (scFOS) is being considered as a possible sweetener for food, because it has a sweet taste. (See the box on page 281, which describes the use of oligosaccharides in infant formula.)

• Inulin is another excellent prebiotic fibre. It's found in many vegetables, but the major sources of inulin in our diet are wheat, onions and green bananas.

How Soluble Fibre Acts as a Prebiotic

The presence of soluble fibre in the gut favours probiotics in two ways. First, fibre helps probiotic microbes to grow. It's also used by non-probiotic microbes, but less effectively. As a result of this difference, the probiotics grow more quickly. Second, as probiotics consume soluble fibre in the intestines, they produce short-chain fatty acids (acids similar to vinegar) as metabolic by-products. The presence of these acids slows the growth of non-probiotic microbes such as *E. coli*. This gives the probiotics an additional competitive advantage.

How Much Fibre Do We Need?

Ideally adults should consume at least 18 grams of fibre per day – or about double the amount in the average UK diet.

Chapter 13 will describe the University of Michigan's Healing Foods Pyramid. If you follow their simple guidelines, you'll automatically get enough fibre. And since all food sources of fibre contain soluble fibre, you'll be supporting the probiotic microbes in your digestive tract.

Sources of Fibre

The usual dietary recommendations don't distinguish between soluble and insoluble fibre. If you're seeking prebiotic benefits, focus on soluble fibre sources. These include oats and oat bran, barley, rice bran, berries, other fruit (unpeeled), vegetables (unpeeled), and legumes (beans, peas and lentils). You won't miss out on insoluble fibre, since the same sources include that, too.

WHAT ABOUT FIBRE SUPPLEMENTS?

It's best to obtain fibre from food rather than from supplements. You'll benefit from all the other healthy nutrients these foods provide – including additional types of prebiotics. Also, food makes it easier to spread your fibre consumption throughout the day, providing probiotic microbes with a continuous source of nourishment.

However, fibre supplements can be valuable for times when your diet is less than ideal. There are a few tips if you're taking a fibre supplement:

• Select a supplement that contains soluble fibre sources, such as FOS, inulin, psyllium, pectin, beta-glucan, guar gum and/or acacia.

• Divide the dose so your gut microbes are nourished throughout the day.

• Drink plenty of water – that helps fibre to do its job.

For a Comfortable Transition

Adding fibre to your diet is a smart move for health. But if you try to make changes too quickly, you may experience temporary gastrointestinal problems, including wind and bloating. This happens because the changes in your microflora aren't keeping up with the improvements in your diet. The temporary result is excess wind production by your gut microbes.

Don't be alarmed if this problem arises – just take it as a signal to slow down. Cut back a little on high-fibre foods until the symptoms go away, then try again. But this time, do it more gradually, so your body has a chance to adjust. Another measure that may help is to increase your consumption of probiotics with a supplement or probiotic shot (see Chapter 11 for recommendations) as you increase your fibre intake.

I want to emphasise that not everyone has these minor difficulties – and when they do occur, they don't last for long. Moreover, many people are delighted by the positive changes fibre can produce. Some find that they no longer need laxatives to stay regular. Others are surprised to discover that they've effortlessly shed a few extra pounds, simply because fibre tames their appetite.

DIETARY PHENOLS

We've all heard the good news about antioxidants – those miraculous compounds that reward us for eating fruit, vegetables and other plant-based foods. Antioxidants are credited with a wide range of dazzling health benefits, from protecting us against cancer to fighting wrinkles. There are lots of different antioxidants, including certain vitamins (beta-carotene, which is a form of vitamin A; vitamin C; and vitamin E). But the most abundant type of antioxidant in plants are compounds called phenols. You've probably heard of many of them: tannins, phytoestrogens, flavonoids, flavonols, bioflavonoids, polyphenols and monophenols. When they are found in food, I refer to them as 'dietary phenols'.

When you eat plant foods rich in phenols, you not only get the familiar benefits of antioxidants, you also support the probiotic microbes in your digestive tract. That's because phenols have the astounding ability to act as selective antibiotics: they inhibit the growth of non-probiotic bacteria, while having minimal effect on the growth of probiotics.

Fighting Oxidation: the Role of Antioxidants

We can't survive without oxygen, but this vital element has a cruel side. Anything exposed to oxygen is vulnerable to oxidation. This damaging chemical process makes metal rust and tarnish; it creates spoilt brown spots on food. And it wreaks slow havoc on our cells.

Oxidative damage in our body can lead to cancer and heart disease; it's also responsible for age-related changes, such as wrinkling of the skin, cataracts and macular degeneration (a leading cause of blindness in the elderly). The cellular damage produced by oxidation stimulates inflammation, creating further problems. Our tissues fight back by producing antioxidants to control oxidation.

Plants also live in a dangerous world. Like us, their enemies include oxidation and harmful microbes. So they do exactly the same thing our bodies do: they manufacture chemicals, including phenols and other antioxidants, to protect themselves. Phenols also have antibiotic properties, so they protect against harmful microbes, too.

By consuming plant-based foods, we gain the additional army of protective compounds they've created. Their dietary phenols now fight our oxidation. Considerable research has linked a diet with abundant plant antioxidants to reduced risk of cancer, cardiovascular disease and stroke, Alzheimer's disease and inflammatory diseases, such as inflammatory bowel disease, asthma and autoimmunity.

The Hidden Factor

When scientists first learnt about these spectacular health effects, we assumed we could ward off the lifelong damage of oxidation by consuming megadoses of antioxidants. But things weren't so simple. We soon learnt that people who take antioxidants as supplements don't reap the same benefits as those who consume an antioxidant-rich diet. For example, people who eat foods rich in beta-carotene have a reduced risk of lung cancer. Hoping to prevent this terrible disease, medical researchers rushed to initiate major studies in which people at high risk for lung cancer took beta-carotene supplements. But to their dismay and bewilderment, none of these investigations found any protective effect.

Why the difference? Most scientists now speculate that the benefit could come from as-yet-unidentified nutrients in fruit and vegetables; or perhaps antioxidants work together, so a single one can't be effective on its own. We favour a completely different explanation: the unrecognised role of dietary phenols and other prebiotics in helping probiotics to tame inflammation.

Foods rich in antioxidants contain not only antioxidant vitamins like beta-carotene; they're also full of dietary phenols and soluble fibre. What's more, these prebiotics don't just fight oxidation, they also inhibit the growth of many non-probiotic microbes in our microflora, while having less impact on probiotics. Antioxidant vitamins may steal the credit, but behind the scenes, potent prebiotics are fostering the probiotics in our gut microflora and thereby controlling inflammation. As new research expands our understanding of inflammation – a process just as devastating as oxidation, but potentially much easier for us to control – we expect the spotlight to shift. Finally, dietary phenols, probiotics and the gut microflora will get the attention they deserve.

Best Food Sources of Dietary Phenols

There's no minimum daily requirement for dietary phenols. No label tells you how much flavonoid, tannin, phytoestrogen or other phenols a food contains. But here's a simple strategy to safely boost your intake of dietary phenols. Simply follow current guidelines for healthy eating – but make choices within those guidelines to optimise phenol consumption. Here are the best sources:

Beans	Tea
Peas	Red wine
Lentils	Red wine vinegar
Herbs and spices	Dark beer (ales and stout)
Fruit (consumed with the skin)	Dark chocolate
Berries	Cocoa powder
Juices of dark berries (unfiltered and unsweetened)	Coffee (limit to 3 cups per day)

Dietary phenols are more heat-stable than probiotics, but less so than fibre. They can be heated briefly above body temperature without breaking down. For example, you can use boiling water to brew tea. However, extended boiling, baking, grilling or frying can dramatically decrease their concentration. (Later in this chapter I'll explain in more detail how to preserve phenol content in cooked foods.)

Fruit and vegetables usually have the highest phenol content and the most flavour when they're fresh. But frozen and dried versions are excellent sources, too. As a rule, you optimise prebiotic value if you consume fruit and vegetables raw. However, there are two exceptions: tomatoes and Chinese cabbages, such as napa and pak choi. For these vegetables, cooking is preferable because heating releases extra dietary phenols.

METABIOTICS

Scientists investigating the health effects of live bacteria in yoghurt sometimes ran into a mysterious phenomenon: killing the bacteria didn't eliminate their benefits. They would set up an experiment in which one group consumed yoghurt kept under constant refrigeration. The control group would get the same yoghurt, but first the researchers heated it to make sure all the bacteria were dead. A third group would receive unfermented milk with no bacteria. The findings would always be the same: live bacteria produced the most benefits; unfermented milk gave the least. But the heated yoghurt fell somewhere in between.

Dead bacteria can't populate the gut and send beneficial signals to the immune system. How could they possibly produce beneficial effects? Some have guessed that dead bacteria adhere to the lining of the gastrointestinal tract, crowding out harmful competitors. But there's another reason. Even if a fermented food no longer contains live bacteria, their metabolic by-products remain. As I explained in Chapter 10, some of these by-products – which I call metabiotics – are good for our health. In addition, some indirectly benefit us because they serve as prebiotics. I'll describe the few we know about, but I suspect that future research might reveal others.

Short-Chain Fatty Acids

The probiotic microflora in your gut use fermentation to break down fibre into nutrients called short-chain fatty acids (SCFAs). Examples are acetic acid (the acid in vinegar), butyric acid and propionic acid. All of these are found in fermented foods.

 THE LONG AND THE SHORT OF FATTY ACIDS

Acetic acid, butyric acid and propionic acid aren't fats. However, they're called short-chain fatty acids because of their chemical structure. A molecule of a fatty acid consists of a chain of carbon atoms attached to hydrogen and oxygen atoms. The carbon chain can be as short as one atom – or as long as nearly thirty atoms. Short-chain fatty acids contain only a few carbon atoms. These substances are soluble in water and we don't normally think of them as fats. More familiar fatty acids, such as polyunsaturated fatty acids, have longer carbon chains.

SCFAs are the single most important type of metabiotic. They contribute to a healthy digestive tract in several ways:

- They create an environment that favours probiotics and thus help to maintain a balanced microflora. *Candida albicans* and other potentially harmful yeasts don't grow well in the presence of SCFAs.
- They nourish the cells that line the colon, promoting the integrity of the intestinal wall. Some scientists believe that a healthy intestinal wall is a key to preventing food allergies, because it keeps digested food from escaping into the body and stimulating an immune reaction.
- They send signals that limit inflammatory responses. Dendritic cells (a type of white blood cell that I described in Chapter 4) live among the cells that line the intestines; they monitor the GI tract for threats. When enough SCFAs are detected, these monitoring cells send an 'all clear' signal to the immune system. This dampens inflammatory responses in the gut and also stimulates formation of regulatory T cells that travel throughout the body, keeping inflammation under control.

Bacteriocins

Bacteriocins are natural antibiotics that bacteria make to help themselves survive. These antibiotics aren't harmful to the bacteria that make them, but they kill or inhibit other bacteria. The bacteriocins produced by probiotic bacteria help to shift the microbial balance in their own favour. Fermented foods – such as yoghurt, cheese, sourdough bread and sauerkraut – contain bacteriocins, thanks to the lactic acid bacteria in them.

Food Sources of Metabiotics

All foods fermented by probiotic bacteria contain metabiotics – even foods that have been heated after fermentation, so that the bacteria themselves are no longer alive. If you cook with yoghurt or kefir, or if you melt aged cheese, the probiotics contained in these foods will die. But their beneficial metabiotics remain. Similarly, when fermented gherkins and sauerkraut are processed with heat to extend their shelf life, they still provide metabiotics. One of my favourite sources of metabiotics is sourdough bread, which is made with a fermented starter culture that includes live bacteria as well as yeast.

MILK PROTEINS

When you consume probiotics in fermented dairy products, you automatically get additional benefits from milk proteins. One nutritional plus is the protein itself. Of course, most of us get plenty of protein in our diets anyway. However, dairy foods package their protein in particularly convenient forms that can be consumed with little or no preparation. In addition, two milk proteins – lactoferrin and GMP – serve as prebiotics.

What if you're lactose intolerant? Don't worry about missing

IMPROVING INFANT FORMULA WITH SOLUBLE FIBRE AND MILK PROTEINS

The microflora of breastfed and bottle-fed babies are different, which may help explain the health advantages of breastfeeding. Some manufacturers have begun to add probiotic bacteria to infant formula – and research suggests that babies benefit. Another promising approach is to add the following prebiotics:

• **Oligosaccharides:** These soluble fibres are a negligible part of cow's milk, but abundant in human breast milk.

• **GMP:** This prebiotic peptide is found in milk and milk curds, but not in whey. Infant formula is commonly whey-based, so it usually lacks GMP.

• **Alpha-lactalbumin:** Between 20 and 25 per cent of the protein in human milk is alpha-lactalbumin; in cow's milk it's only 2 to 5 per cent. Studies suggest that as a baby digests alpha-lactalbumin, beneficial peptides form temporarily and act against harmful bacteria. This could help to explain why breastfeeding offers protection against infection.

When babies consume formula in which these prebiotics are adjusted to match human breast milk, they develop a microflora that's high in *Bifidobacterium* and otherwise similar to that of breastfed babies. The hope is that these changes will also duplicate the health advantages that breastfeeding provides.

At the moment, probiotic- and prebiotic-enriched baby formulas are available only from speciality sources. But they're expected to hit supermarket shelves in the near future, probably with advertising fanfare and prominent labels.

out. These prebiotics aren't as significant for our microflora as soluble fibre or dietary phenols, and some of the same benefits are available from non-dairy foods. But if you enjoy yoghurt, kefir and cultured cheese, add milk proteins to the list of reasons these foods are good for you.

Lactoferrin

Lactoferrin is a milk protein that binds iron. (The name comes from the Latin words *lac* for 'milk' and *ferrum* for 'iron'.) The microbes that live inside us – good and bad – compete for available iron, because they all need iron to grow. Lactoferrin is an ally to probiotic bacteria in this competition, since it binds the iron in milk very tightly. Probiotic bacteria can strip off the iron, but many non-probiotic bacteria can't. This gives probiotics a growth advantage.

GMP (Glycomacropeptide)

GMP is a fragment of casein, a milk protein. As milk is digested, its proteins break down; protein fragments, called peptides, are released into the gastrointestinal tract. One such peptide is GMP. Research suggests that it inhibits the ability of harmful bacteria to adhere to cells in the intestinal lining. If a microbe can't stick to these cells, it's at a competitive disadvantage. Since probiotic microbes aren't inhibited in this way by GMP, it favours the growth of probiotics.

Making the Most of Milk Proteins

High heat destroys the prebiotic capabilities of milk proteins, though not their nutritional value. So if you scald milk to make a cup of hot chocolate, forget about the lactoferrin and GMP. But these prebiotics are a bonus in yoghurt, kefir, cheeses and any other dairy products that undergo processing at lower temperatures, including pasteurisation.

⚡ FOODS TO AVOID ⚡

You – and your gut microflora – are what you eat. Just as consuming plenty of probiotics and prebiotics promotes a microfloral balance favourable to good health, other foods give the advantage to harmful microbes. Refined carbohydrates – which have lost fibre and other nutrients during processing – are the ones to avoid, or at least to minimise. These include foods like white rice and anything made from white flour rather than wholewheat flour. The ultimate refined carbohydrate is sugar, whose calories are described as 'empty' because they lack added nutritional value.

Refining grains removes valuable components, including dietary phenols, vitamins and minerals, as well as fibre. Although dietary fibre helps probiotics to compete in the gut, some studies find that refined carbohydrates favour the growth of non-probiotic microbes. Refined carbohydrate products – such as bread made from white flour – may be enriched to restore selected nutrients. But enrichment seldom restores fibre and phenols.

Whenever possible, choose whole grains instead of refined ones. That means substituting whole grain bread for white bread, brown rice for white rice, wholewheat pasta for white pasta and whole grain breakfast cereals for the sugar-coated refined varieties. If you don't want to eliminate sugar completely, try to cut back gradually. The more can reduce your intake of refined carbohydrates, the more favourable the environment you create for the probiotics that live in your digestive tract.

POLYUNSATURATED FATTY ACIDS

In the 1980s and 1990s, fat was a despised nutrient. Non-fat foods – some loaded with ingredients that were at least as unwholesome – ruled supermarket shelves, promising weight loss and good health simply because of what they *didn't* contain. Today our view of fat is more nuanced. Some fats – the saturated ones and trans fats – can indeed be harmful to health if consumption isn't limited. But other fats are actually good for us.

The healthiest diets, we now know, are not ones that are fat-free, but ones in which the fats are mostly unsaturated rather than saturated. The Mediterranean diet is one example. And guess what: one type of good-for-us fat is a prebiotic.

The fat in food and in our bodies is made up of molecules called fatty acids. Evidence from animal studies suggests that some of these – the polyunsaturated fatty acids (PUFAs) – may act as prebiotics. However, it's clear that the prebiotic value of PUFAs is not as important as that of fibre and dietary phenols. And we're a long way from knowing exactly how much we'd need to consume to make a meaningful difference in our gut microflora. Nevertheless, the prebiotic value of PUFAs offers added motivation to balance our fat consumption in favour of unsaturated fats.

A QUICK GUIDE TO FATS

Fatty acids, the building blocks of fat, are classified as saturated, monounsaturated or polyunsaturated. All fats contain a combination of these three types; their properties are determined by the fatty acid that predominates. In addition, manufacturers can create trans fats by adding hydrogen to liquid fats.

TYPE OF FAT	EFFECTS ON HEALTH	HOW TO IDENTIFY	FOOD SOURCES
Polyunsaturated	Reduces the risk of heart disease and stroke	Liquid at room temperature; remains liquid when chilled	Corn oil, rapeseed oil, soya bean oil and oily fish such as salmon, tuna and herring
Monounsaturated	Lowers cardiovascular risk	Liquid at room temperature; thickens when chilled	Olive oil, rapeseed oil, peanut oil, avocado, olives, nuts
Saturated	Linked to risk of cardiovascular disease	Solid at room temperature	Meat, butter and other dairy foods, cocoa butter, palm oil, coconut oil
Trans fat	Linked to risk of cardiovascular disease	Solid at room temperature	Processed foods, including vegetable shortening, biscuits, snacks

MY TOP TEN LIST

Even if you're already nutrition-conscious, selecting foods for their prebiotic content involves a slight shift in focus. This section highlights ten personal favourites – delicious foods that contain notable quantities of the prebiotics mentioned in this chapter. Some are already familiar – but you might need to eat or prepare them a little differently to maximise their prebiotic benefit. Others may not yet be part of your daily diet, but I hope you'll be tempted to try them.

Fruit and Vegetables – Including the Skins

If your mother told you that the skins of fruit and vegetables were the healthiest part, she was right. Phenols are found just under the skin of fruit and vegetables, where they can ward off invaders that land on their surfaces. In addition to phenols, fruit and vegetables supply soluble fibre plus many important vitamins and minerals.

The dietary phenol powerhouses are berries: blueberries, raspberries, cranberries, blackberries and strawberries. That's because berries have the highest ratio of skin to pulp. Similarly, cherries – especially tart red cherries (the kind most often used to make pie filling) – also are unusually high in dietary phenols.

Trail Mix: A Prebiotic Convenience Food

This delicious blend of nuts, seeds and dried fruit isn't just for hikes! Trail mix is equally nutritious and convenient when you're at home or at work. Nuts and seeds are great sources of fibre, plus protein and dietary phenols. Dried fruit has lost much of its water, but not its phenols and fibre.

Make your own trail mix, or buy it ready-made. A few tips for creating or selecting a nutritious blend:

• Avoid mixes that contain sweets or yoghurt-covered nuts, since both add a significant amount of refined sugar.
• Look for unblanched nuts. Blanching removes the papery brown skin that surrounds and protects the nut – and that's where the health-promoting phenols are concentrated.
• Favour dried fruit without added sugar; it's sometimes easier to find in a health food store.

Kids love trail mix. Add it to cereals, yoghurt and salads. Or eat it as an instant meal or snack when you're on the move – trail mix travels well, because it doesn't require refrigeration. Note: nuts, seeds and dried fruit are concentrated foods, so watch portion size. A little goes a long way.

Dark Berry Juices

Certain fruit juices are excellent sources of dietary phenols – but they must be carefully selected.

• Look for juices made from blueberries, raspberries, blackberries, blackcurrants, cranberries, pomegranates, tart cherries and Concord grapes. Processing these fruit into juice reduces their dietary phenol content, but significant levels remain.
• Choose dark juices. In general, juices that you can't see through are higher in dietary phenols than clear juices.
• Check the sugar content, especially for juice blends and juice drinks. Often the primary ingredient is either sugar water or a clear juice like apple, white grape or pear – juices that are low in dietary phenols and full of sugar, even if it comes from fruit. One exception is cranberry juice cocktail. A one-to-one mix of juice and sugar water is less tart than pure cranberry juice, but the cocktail is still loaded with dietary phenols. By the way, a splash of a dark berry juice adds a touch of sweetness and flavour to tea or plain tonic water.

Herbs and Spices

Herbs and spices are an unappreciated source of phenols in the diet. Their intense flavour comes from the same phenols found in the skin of fruit and vegetables, but in far more concentrated form. If you put a pinch of a herb or spice on your tongue, you can taste the characteristic bitterness of the phenols it contains.

Just about every herb and spice tested has been found to contain significant amounts of dietary phenols – but oregano tops the list. This popular herb, familiar to anyone who loves pizza, boasts one of the highest phenol contents of any food. Fresh spices and herbs have more dietary phenols than dried versions. But as long as the flavour is strong, the phenols are still there.

When you sprinkle chopped fresh herbs and spices on food, you reap the full benefits. But some strategic planning is required when you cook. Here's the underlying issue: if herbs and spices are briefly boiled in liquid, their phenols are extracted. But if this phenol-rich fluid simmers for a long time – or if herbs and spices are cooked at high temperature – these valuable compounds lose much of their prebiotic value. To optimise both flavour and phenol benefit, add herbs and spices in two stages to soups, casseroles and other dishes that involve heat: at the beginning, so that the flavour will permeate the dish, and again just before serving, to deliver phenols.

Since phenols are more easily extracted from herbs and spices by alcohol and oil rather than water, here's another option: purée the herbs and spices in a small amount of red or white wine, and then add some olive oil. Just before serving, stir this mixture into warm sauces. Several of the recipes in Chapter 16 use this technique, which dramatically enhances flavours while maintaining a high prebiotic content.

THE ANTIMICROBIAL POWER OF GARLIC AND MUSTARD

Garlic and mustard seed don't contain phenols. Nor are they prebiotics: though both act as antimicrobials, they don't favour probiotic bacteria. But in combination with a diet high in probiotics, garlic and mustard can help promote a balanced gut microflora by making room for a strong infusion of probiotic bacteria.

Whole Grain Sourdough Bread

Wheat flour naturally contains lactic acid bacteria and a variety of yeasts. When flour is mixed with water and the resulting batter is left in a warm place, it usually begins to ferment. After a few days, the batter is ready to use as a starter to make bread dough. (Some of this starter can be saved and added to a new batch of flour and water to speed the process the next time.) Until the mid-nineteenth century, all leavened bread was prepared with a starter culture.

The yeast in the starter produces carbon dioxide gas, which makes the bread dough rise. The characteristically tart taste of sourdough bread comes from the acids produced by the starter's lactic acid bacteria. Though the bacteria die during baking, they leave behind healthy – and flavourful – metabiotics, including short-chain fatty acids and bacteriocins.

Packaged yeast simplifies bread making: a starter culture isn't needed and the results are more reliable as well as faster. But ordinary yeast breads don't contain the metabiotics that sourdough provides, nor can they match the flavour.

I hope you'll get acquainted with sourdough bread. When you buy it, look for the words 'culture' or 'starter' on the label, to make sure that the sour taste is produced by fermentation. Any sourdough supplies valuable metabiotics – but if you select whole grain bread, it delivers fibre, too.

Oats

Oats are loaded with beta-glucan, a form of soluble fibre that acts as a prebiotic. Oatmeal was the first whole food that the Food and Drug Administration permitted to make a health claim on the label: 'Soluble fibre from oatmeal, as part of a diet low in saturated fat and cholesterol, may reduce the risk of heart disease.'

In today's hectic world, many of us are less familiar with

old-fashioned oatmeal, or porridge, than with the instant version or with oat-containing muesli and cold cereals. Oatmeal, or porridge, has excellent nutritional value, whether it's the old-fashioned kind, quick or instant. However, be aware that instant oatmeal packets are usually loaded with sugar. If you choose a plain version, you can easily add your own flavourings: dried fruit, chopped nuts, cinnamon and a small amount of sugar, honey or golden syrup if sweetness is desired. Many people prefer the chewy texture of old-fashioned rolled or steel-cut oats, but assume they take too much time to prepare. However, it's easy to cook porridge in a microwave.

Porridge isn't just a superb breakfast food. You can substitute rolled oats for breadcrumbs in many foods, and use rolled oats instead of wheat flour for crumb toppings on pies, muffins and cakes.

Legumes

Legumes – such as beans, lentils and peanuts – are loaded with soluble fibre and dietary phenols, not to mention protein and minerals. These are versatile, convenient and healthy foods, and most of us would do well to eat more of them.

The dietary phenol content of beans is one of the highest per weight of any food. In general, the darker the colour of the bean, the higher the phenol content. That's great news for anyone who enjoys black beans as much as I do. A few simple tips for adding beans and lentils to your diet:

• Substitute legumes for all or part of the meat in your usual recipes for soups, casseroles and pasta sauces.
• Add cooked beans to salads.
• Purée beans into spreads, such as garlicky hummus, which can serve as dips or sandwich fillings.

Though the name suggests otherwise, peanuts are actually a legume rather than a nut. They're an excellent source of protein and dietary phenols – and the phenol content is even higher if they're roasted. To get the full prebiotic advantage, be sure to consume the papery outer layer of the nut. This is often discarded in processing or when you crack open the shell, but that's where the phenols are concentrated. Spanish peanuts – my personal favourite – rival apples and carrots for phenol content. Also, keep in mind that peanuts contain more fat than other legumes, and adjust portions accordingly.

Tea

Aside from water, tea is the healthiest drink on the planet. Dietary phenols are extracted from the leaves during brewing, giving the beverage an exceptionally high phenol content. Just think: all those phenols and no calories (when drunk without milk)! Numerous studies have shown that regular consumption of tea reduces heart attacks.

To fully extract the phenols, tea must be brewed with boiling water. Once it's brewed, it can be served hot or cold. Because phenols don't dissolve well in cold water, 'refrigerator' and 'sun' tea, which are prepared from cool or room-temperature water, don't provide these valuable nutrients. Incidentally, low phenol content is what gives these teas a smooth taste – phenols are bitter-tasting. If you find that regular tea is too bitter, dilute it with water, or add berry juice or lemon juice and a small amount of sugar.

Green tea has the highest phenol content; black tea is a close second. (Though coffee contains some phenols, it's far behind.) Both green and black tea contain caffeine. If you prefer to limit caffeine, select a version of regular tea that's been decaffeinated with carbon dioxide, the gas used to make carbonated drinks (the process is sometimes called effervescent decaffeination). Another natural and non-toxic solvent used for decaffeination is ethyl acetate, which is found in many plant products. However, this can remove more of the phenols and leave an aftertaste. Tea decaffeinated with carbon dioxide has only half the phenol content of regular tea, but it's still a good source. In contrast, these valuable prebiotics are not found in herbal teas or instant teas.

Red Wine

Moderate consumption of red wine – a glass or two per day – has been linked to reduced risk for cardiovascular disease and other health benefits, thanks to the antioxidants it contains. And I'm sure you've heard about one particular antioxidant found in red wine, resveratrol. Many scientists believe that the resveratrol in wine helps explain why the incidence of heart disease is relatively low in France, despite a cuisine that's rich in cream and butter.

Now you have yet another reason to enjoy wine with dinner: prebiotics. Red wine has one of the highest phenol contents of any food or beverage. That's because it's made not only with the pulp of the grapes, but also with the crushed skins and seeds. (White wine uses only the pulp.) As yeast ferments the grapes' sugars to make wine, alcohol is produced. The phenols in the fruit skins and seeds dissolve more readily in alcohol than in water, so these valuable compounds are even more concentrated in wine than in plain juice made from the same grapes.

Dark Chocolate and Cocoa Powder

I'm delighted to report that dark chocolate and cocoa powder are excellent sources of dietary phenols. (Skip milk chocolate if you're looking for prebiotics, because its processing decreases the phenol content.) The higher the cocoa content of the chocolate, the higher the phenol content. Some chocolates don't list the proportion of cocoa on the label, but speciality and imported chocolates often do.

Another way to identify a phenol-rich chocolate is by its flavour. Phenols are bitter-tasting, so the richest sources are dark, bittersweet chocolates. Savour the intensity so that a modest portion satisfies you.

Adding prebiotics to my own diet has been much more of a pleasure than a chore. And it's been surprisingly easy to convince my kids to do the same. I hope you and your family enjoy these healthy foods as much as we do. *Bon appétit!*

CHAPTER THIRTEEN

A Comprehensive Food Plan for Good Health

In 2002, when I decided to add probiotics and prebiotics to my diet, I wasn't following any particular food plan. But I liked the idea of making dietary changes within a nutritionally sound framework. I was focused on one health goal, namely reducing my allergy and asthma symptoms. However, I didn't want to lose track of other important dietary objectives, such as minimising my risk of heart disease and cancer.

Colleagues had recently developed the University of Michigan Healing Foods Pyramid. Their guidelines, which share features with the USDA Food Guide Pyramid and the Harvard Healthy Eating Pyramid, made sense to me. So I used them as a basis for my new way of eating. Within this framework, I made food choices to emphasise probiotics and prebiotics. As a result, my diet was automatically healthy overall.

This chapter describes relevant parts of the Healing Foods Pyramid and explains how to use them to promote a healthy microflora. These particular guidelines aren't the only ones you can use. The same approach works with any flexible plan for healthy eating, including weight loss programmes like Weight Watchers and the South Beach Diet.

THE UNIVERSITY OF MICHIGAN HEALING FOODS PYRAMID

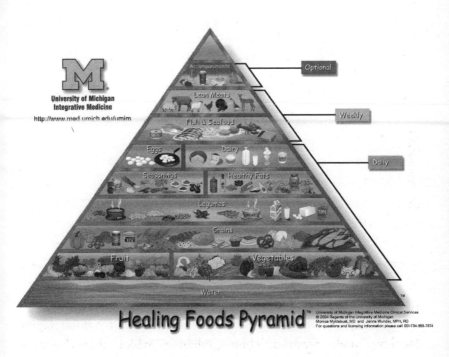

Healing Foods Pyramid

The Healing Foods Pyramid was created by Monica Myklebust, MD, and Jenna Wunder, MPH, RD, at the University of Michigan's Department of Family Medicine. They included only foods known to have essential nutrients or other healing benefits. (I was pleased to learn that this concept was broad enough to include dark chocolate.) At the base of the pyramid are plant foods. Animal foods can be added or omitted, as you wish. The Pyramid celebrates the pleasure of eating, with a tempting array of colours and textures and the advice to savour and enjoy your food.

You can learn more about the Healing Foods Pyramid by visiting the website of the University of Michigan Integrative Medicine: http://www.med.umich.edu/umim. Excerpts are included below with the permission of the copyright holders, the Regents of the University of Michigan, Monica Myklebust, MD, and Jenna Wunder, MPH, RD.

NOURISHING OURSELVES – AND OUR MICROFLORA

The University of Michigan Healing Foods Pyramid offers ample choices. I'll go through the relevant food groups and explain how to work within their guidelines to maximise consumption of probiotics and prebiotics.

Dairy

Before probiotics became a consideration, the only dairy food I consumed daily was the milk I added to my coffee. As far as I was concerned, dairy foods were just another source of protein, and I had plenty of other protein in my diet. But once I realised the importance of probiotics, fermented dairy products took centre stage.

I now look forward to my daily breakfast of yoghurt, muesli and fruit. Yoghurt, kefir and cheese are my favourite snacks, and I often fit them into lunch and dinner, too. Out of curiosity, I once tried replacing the milk in my coffee with a scoop of yoghurt. One sip put an end to that experiment! But other than a small amount of milk for coffee, all the dairy food I consume is fermented.

Probiotics and protein aren't the only valuable nutrients found in these foods. They're among the richest sources of calcium and other minerals the body needs, and are also high in vitamin B_{12}. True, most dairy foods contain saturated fat. However, you can maintain control of fat and calories by consuming low-fat and non-fat versions.

To make sure you get plenty of probiotics, select fermented dairy products. The best sources are yoghurt and kefir (check the label to make sure they contain live cultures) and aged cheese. See the tables that follow for serving sizes.

Though the Pyramid guidelines warn that full-fat cheese is high in saturated fat, they also note that small amounts can be an important dietary component. All of the cheeses in the table overleaf contain probiotics.

University of Michigan Healing Foods Pyramid
SELECTED LOW-FAT AND NON-FAT DAIRY SOURCES
1 to 3 servings per day (optional)

LOW-FAT OR NON-FAT DAIRY FOOD (LESS THAN 3 GRAMS OF FAT PER SERVING)	SERVING SIZE
Yoghurt	8 ounces, or 230 grams
Frozen yoghurt	8 ounces, or 230 grams
Cottage cheese	4 ounces, or 110 grams
Cream cheese	1 tablespoon
Sour cream	2 tablespoons
Semi-skimmed ricotta cheese	1 ounce or 30 grams
Semi-skimmed mozzarella	30 grams
Skimmed milk (up to 1% fat)	240 ml

University of Michigan Healing Foods Pyramid
FULL-FAT CHEESES
Up to 1 serving per day (optional). Serving size: 30 to 60 grams

Soft	Brie, Mascarpone
Semi-hard	Blue, Feta
Hard	Cheddar, Swiss
Very hard	Parmesan, Romano

Some people are lactose intolerant: they can't digest lactose, the sugar found in milk. A less common problem is sensitivity to casein, a milk protein. For these reasons, the Healing Foods Pyramid makes dairy optional. As explained on page 226 in Chapter 10, some lactose intolerant individuals can digest fermented dairy products.

If you can't tolerate or don't enjoy dairy foods, you can find most of the same nutrients elsewhere. Though it's difficult to get sufficient probiotics without dairy, there are other options. One is soya yoghurt (see 'Legumes' section of this chapter); another is probiotic supplements (see Chapter 11).

Fruit and Vegetables

Do I need to mention that fruit and vegetables are good for you? I'm sure you know that they're excellent sources of fibre, and also rich in vitamins and minerals. Scientists have identified thousands of other health-promoting phytochemicals (i.e., chemical substances found in plants). One fruit or vegetable may contain a hundred different phytochemicals. In addition to all their other valuable nutrients, fruit and vegetables offer prebiotics. Among these are soluble fibre and dietary phenols, a group of phytochemicals. It's not quite clear which specific substances deserve the credit, but considerable research evidence shows that the more fruit and vegetables you eat, the less likely you are to develop a chronic disease.

Some people are dismayed to learn that it takes at least seven servings per day to make a difference. This reaction explains why I don't like the term 'serving'. It makes me think of what my mum put on my plate when I was growing up. Those were double-sized portions! But the Healing Foods Pyramid, which suggests seven to ten servings of fruit and vegetables daily, is talking about a modest amount per serving – for example, just six or seven baby carrots, or an apple the size of a tennis ball, which is only 6–7 cm in diameter.

If you tuck lettuce and tomato slices into a sandwich, that's a vegetable serving. And if your apple is large (i.e. about 8 cm in diameter), it counts as two servings of fruit.

University of Michigan Integrative Medicine Healing Foods Pyramid SELECTED FRUIT AND VEGETABLES 7 to 10 servings per day	
FRUIT OR VEGETABLE	SERVING SIZE
Raw leafy greens	8 ounces, or 230 grams
Baby carrots	6 to 7
Apple or orange	Size of tennis ball
Banana	Medium
Grapes	17
Berries	170 grams
Melon, chopped	8 ounces, or 230 grams
Raw, chopped fruit or vegetables	4 ounces, or 110 grams
Cooked vegetables	4 ounces, or 110 grams
Dried fruit	2 ounces, or 60 grams

Don't overlook fermented vegetables, which offer probiotics, prebiotics and metabiotics, as well as all the other benefits. Count the following as a single vegetable serving – and feel free to take seconds, because they're low in calories: 110 grams of sauerkraut or kimchi, 110 grams of fermented gherkin slices or half of a deli-style gherkin.

The Pyramid doesn't recommend drinking juices, because they usually lack the fibre of whole fruit and are high in calories. It's true that most juices are filtered. That's why they're clear enough to see through. Some clear juices – like apple, pear and white grape – which can be found on their own or used in juice blends, are high in sugar and have little or no dietary phenols. However, the following unfiltered juices are valuable enough for their phenol content that I recommend including unsweetened versions in a healthy diet: pomegranate, blackcurrant, Concord grape, cranberry, blueberry, blackberry, tart cherry and raspberry. But even the unsweetened versions are high in sugar. For that reason, restrict them to one serving per day.

When you plan menus or reach for a snack, try to emphasise fruit and vegetables that offer soluble fibre and phenols. Some of the best sources of these prebiotics are:

Sources of Soluble Fibre	*Sources of Dietary Phenols*
Fruit, consumed with the skin	Fruit, consumed with the skin
Berries	Berries
Vegetables, unpeeled	Selected juices: pomegranate, blackcurrant, Concord grape, cranberry, blueberry, blackberry, tart cherry, and raspberry (unfiltered and unsweetened)

Grains and Starchy Vegetables

Grains and starchy vegetables are the staple foods of every cuisine. They're sometimes referred to as the staff of life because their carbohydrates supply most of the body's energy needs. Starchy vegetables – such as sweetcorn, potatoes, squash, plantains and the harder-to-find yucca (cassava root) – aren't grains. But the body metabolises them as if they were grains rather than vegetables. Like grains, they provide ample fibre and nutrients.

For optimal health benefits, the Healing Foods Pyramid recommends whole grains rather than milled, processed or refined grains. As the name implies, whole grains contain the entire grain. They're loaded with soluble and insoluble fibre, as well as essential vitamins and minerals, including the B vitamins, vitamin E, folate, selenium and more. In contrast, refined grains lose both the bran and the germ – and all the nutrients they contain. Processed versions of these grains are often 'enriched', which means that some of the lost nutrients are added back. However, enrichment doesn't restore all the nutrients; nor is the fibre returned.

All foods that contain fibre have both the soluble and the insoluble kind. But some have more of one than the other. Remember that only soluble fibre offers prebiotic benefits. So when you select grains, include ones that are particularly rich in soluble fibre: oats, brown rice and barley.

Whole grains can take some getting used to. They may taste slightly bitter because of the phenols they contain, and their texture is crunchier. I've found that once I made the change, though, I actually preferred them.

One of my family's favourite sources of whole grains is muesli. But you have to check the label before you buy. Some commercial mueslis are as sweet and rich as biscuits. However, others are packed with flavourful, nutritious grains and are low in fat and sugar. I eat muesli with yoghurt and fruit for breakfast nearly every day.

Legumes: Beans, Peas, Lentils and Soya

Legumes are prebiotic powerhouses, with high levels of dietary phenols and soluble fibre. In addition, they're excellent sources of low-fat protein with the bonuses of antioxidants, iron, zinc, calcium, selenium and folate.

University of Michigan Healing Foods Pyramid
SELECTED WHOLE GRAINS AND STARCHY VEGETABLES
4 to 11 servings per day

WHOLE GRAINS AND STARCHY VEGETABLES	SERVING SIZE
Wholewheat or whole grain bread	1 slice (30 grams)
Brown rice, millet, quinoa, barley or polenta	80 grams
Wholewheat couscous	80 grams
Wholewheat or multigrain pasta	80 grams
Whole grain crackers and pretzels	20 grams
Tortilla chips	20 grams
Potato with skin	1 medium
Wholewheat or whole grain bagel, 110 grams	¼
Whole grain pancake or waffle, 10 cm across	1
Wholewheat pitta, 15 cm across	½
Porridge; cooked cereal based on barley or bran	170 grams

Despite their favourable nutrition profile, I used to avoid beans. I liked the flavour, but not the gassy consequences. (There's a reason they're popularly known as the 'musical fruit'.) It didn't occur to me that my body could adjust to them, but it has – thanks to the new balance of bacteria in my gut. I now enjoy beans in many forms – hummus, soups, sauces, stews and chilli. I particularly like black beans, which have a rich, beefy flavour.

If you eat meat and poultry more than once or twice a week, consider substituting legumes at least some of the time. When you introduce them gradually, you're much less likely to experience wind. Also, if you like yoghurt, try soya yoghurt – it provides the same probiotics as conventional yoghurt, plus the prebiotics in soya. This is an especially valuable option if you're sensitive to dairy foods.

Healthy Fats

All fats are not created equal. As I explained in Chapter 12, some are actually good for us. The Healing Foods Pyramid recommends fats that consist mainly of monounsaturated fatty acids or that contain a type of polyunsaturated fatty acids called omega-3. The guidelines suggest limiting saturated fats and trans fats. (Trans fats are found in liquid vegetable oils that have been chemically processed with hydrogen so that they're solid at room temperature. If you see 'hydrogenated' or 'partially hydrogenated' vegetable oils on the label, the food contains trans fats.)

These days, my favourite sources of fat are nuts and extra virgin or virgin olive oil. We dip bread into olive oil instead of using butter. I enjoy its delicate flavour even more because of the dietary phenols it contains. Nuts and seeds – as well as butters made from them – are excellent sources of healthy monounsaturated fats. Both have additional prebiotic value because of their fibre and dietary phenols.

University of Michigan Healing Foods Pyramid
SELECTED LEGUMES
1 to 3 servings per day

TYPES	SERVING SIZE
Beans	
Chickpeas, lima beans, fava beans, black beans, black-eyed peas, kidney beans, navy beans, great northern beans, pinto beans, adzuki beans, mung beans	110 grams tinned or cooked

80 grams mashed |
Peas	
Split, yellow or green	
Lentils	
Large or small; brown, green, red or black	
Soya (1 to 2 servings per day)	
Soya beans (edamamé)	110 grams, cooked
Miso soup	110 grams
Soya milk	240 ml
Soya nuts	28 grams
Soya yoghurt	240 ml
Tempeh	110 grams
Tofu	110 grams

University of Michigan Healing Foods Pyramid
SELECTED HEALTHY FATS
3 to 9 servings per day

OILS (serving size is 1 teaspoon)	NUTS (SERVING SIZE)	SEEDS (SERVING SIZE)	BUTTERS (SERVING SIZE)	OTHER (SERVING SIZE)
Olive oil	Macadamias (2 to 3)	Sesame seeds (1 tablespoon)	Almond butter (½ tablespoon)	Avocado (2 tablespoons or 1 ounce)
Rapeseed oil	Hazelnuts (5)	Pumpkin seeds (47 seeds)	Cashew butter (½ tablespoon)	Black olives (8)
Peanut oil	Pecans (5 halves)	Ground flaxseed (1 tablespoon)	Peanut butter (½ tablespoon)	Green olives (10)
Sesame oil	Almonds (7)	Sunflower seeds (3 tablespoons)	Tahini or sesame paste (2 teaspoons)	
Walnut oil	Cashews (6)		Sunflower seed butter (2 teaspoons)	
Soya bean oil	Pistachios (17)			
Grape seed oil	Brazil nuts (2)			
Flaxseed oil (should be consumed raw and not used in cooking)	Peanuts (9)			
	Pine nuts (50)			
	Walnuts (4 halves)			

Polyunsaturated fatty acids (PUFAs) also may have prebiotic activity. Omega-3 fatty acids, a type of PUFA, help to prevent overexuberant inflammatory responses in the body. Some research suggests that omega-3s also help prevent and treat heart disease, high blood pressure, inflammation, mental health disorders, diabetes, digestive disorders, autoimmune disease and cancer – a remarkable list. The richest sources of these prebiotic fats are fatty fish (see the next section). However, they're also found in certain plant foods.

University of Michigan Healing Foods Pyramid SELECTED PLANT SOURCES OF OMEGA-3 FATTY ACIDS (listed from highest to lowest omega-3 content)	
OILS (serving size is 1 teaspoon)	NUTS AND SEEDS (SERVING SIZE)
Flaxseed oil*	Flaxseeds (1 tablespoon)
Walnut oil	Walnuts (4 halves)
Rapeseed oil	Pecans (5 halves)
Soya bean oil	Pine nuts (50)
*Should be consumed raw and not used in cooking.	

Fish and Seafood

These foods are optional but recommended in the Healing Foods Pyramid. Fish and seafood provide iron and vitamin B_{12}, as well as protein. Certain fish – particularly fatty fish that live in cold water – also contain omega-3 fatty acids. If you like fish and seafood, aim for two to four servings per week. Try to include at least two servings of fish with high omega-3 content, shown in the table below.

University of Michigan Healing Foods Pyramid
FISH HIGH IN OMEGA-3 FATTY ACIDS
(2 grams or more per 170-gram serving)

FISH	GRAMS OF OMEGA-3 PER PORTION
Wild salmon	3.2
Pacific and jack mackerel	3.2
Sable fish	3.0
Whitefish	3.0
Pacific sardine	2.8
Bluefin tuna	2.8
Atlantic herring	2.4
Atlantic mackerel	2.0
Rainbow trout	2.0

Seasonings

I think of herbs and spices as vitamins that taste good. All of them, especially oregano, are loaded with dietary phenols. The Healing Foods Pyramid suggests using a variety of spices, herbs and alliums (bulbous plants, such as garlic and chives), and recommends experimenting with hot peppers – but cautiously. As long as you enjoy the flavour, you really can't overdo seasonings. Remember to check the label: artificial and natural flavourings may provide the taste of herbs and spices, but they don't have the prebiotic content.

Accompaniments

Each of the following three accompaniments – tea, alcoholic beverages and dark chocolate – has distinct healing benefits. And that doesn't count how good they taste.

Tea

I've always liked iced tea – and now I have good reasons to drink it year-round. Teas are rich in polyphenols, a type of dietary phenol and antioxidant. The Healing Foods Pyramid suggests two to four cups of tea per day. If you need to limit caffeine, select a decaffeinated tea made with the carbon dioxide (effervescent) process. Note that herbal teas do not contain polyphenols.

Alcoholic Beverages

Research links moderate alcohol consumption to significant health benefits, including lower risk of coronary artery disease, heart attack and stroke. Red wine and dark beers (ales and stouts) are especially good choices, since they provide prebiotics as well as alcohol. Lift a glass at dinner to the health of your gut microbes.

Dark Chocolate

I've saved the best for last: chocolate. Yes, dark chocolate – bitter-sweet or semi-sweet – is a health food. It contains flavonoids (a type of dietary phenol with beneficial antioxidant as well as prebiotic effects) plus a number of minerals, including calcium, magnesium and potassium. According to studies summarised in the Healing Foods Pyramid, chocolate decreases the oxidative effects of LDL (bad) cholesterol, reduces the risk of blood clots, increases blood flow in arteries and may lower high blood pressure. Plus, chocolate may improve mood and pleasure by boosting serotonin and endorphin levels in the brain. That could explain why we like it so much.

University of Michigan Healing Foods Pyramid
SELECTED ALCOHOL BEVERAGE SOURCES

Up to 1 serving per day for women and people over 60;

up to 2 servings per day for men, but no more than 1 per hour*

TYPE OF DRINK	SERVING SIZE
Beer	350 ml
Wine	150 ml
Spirits (whisky, vodka, rum, gin, scotch)	50 ml

* Alcohol consumption is not recommended for:

- Women who are pregnant or planning to become pregnant
- People who plan to drive or engage in other activities that require attention or skill
- People taking medications that interact with alcohol, including some over-the-counter medications
- Individuals with a history of alcoholism or alcohol abuse
- Those under the age of 18

Abstinent individuals should not begin to drink solely for health benefits. Some benefits can be achieved from foods, including grapes or grape juice, instead of alcohol.

The Healing Foods Pyramid suggests an average of 30 grams per day of dark chocolate, or up to 200 grams per week. Select a chocolate that contains 70 per cent or more cocoa solids; avoid those made with hydrogenated or partially hydrogenated oils, which can raise cholesterol. Eat slowly and savour!

When I adopted this healthier way of eating, I knew it would be good for me. But what I wasn't expecting was how much more I would enjoy my new diet. The food I eat now tastes better; the flavours seem more vivid. Perhaps that's in part because I use more herbs and spices. But it's probably also because I've cut back on sugar and have developed an appreciation for bitter tastes.

Food has become more fun for our family. We're more adventurous about trying new things. When we have a chance to browse in the supermarket, it's like a treasure hunt. Another surprise is how much less time my wife and I spend on food preparation. When you know that your fridge is stocked with wholesome food, there's no guilt in grabbing several containers, putting them on the table and declaring that dinner is served. My family's cuisine was never complicated. But it's even simpler now. In the chapters to come, I'll describe some of our short cuts and share our favourite recipes.

MAKING PROBIOTIC AND PREBIOTIC SELECTIONS
WITH THE UNIVERSITY OF MICHIGAN HEALING FOODS PYRAMID

HEALING FOODS PYRAMID FOOD CATEGORY	RECOMMENDED SERVINGS	BEST PROBIOTIC AND PREBIOTIC CHOICES
Dairy	1 to 3 per day	Yoghurt with live cultures Kefir with live cultures Aged cheese
Fruit and vegetables	7 to 10 per day	Vegetables, unpeeled Fermented vegetables Fruit, consumed with the skin Berries Selected juices: pomegranate, blackcurrants, Concord grape, cranberry, blueberry, blackberry, tart cherry and raspberry (unfiltered and unsweetened)
Grains and starchy vegetables	4 to 11 per day	Oats, oatmeal Brown rice Barley
Legumes	1 to 3 per day	All legumes

HEALING FOODS PYRAMID FOOD CATEGORY	RECOMMENDED SERVINGS	BEST PROBIOTIC AND PREBIOTIC CHOICES
Healthy fats	3 to 9 per day	Nuts (especially walnuts, pecans, pine nuts) Seeds (especially flaxseeds) Flaxseed, walnut, rapeseed and soya bean oils
Fish and seafood	2 to 4 per week	Wild salmon, Pacific and jack mackerel, sable fish, whitefish, Pacific sardine, bluefin tuna, Atlantic herring, Atlantic mackerel, rainbow trout
Seasonings	Use liberally	Oregano and other herbs and spices
Tea	2 to 4 cups per day	Regular tea or tea decaffeinated with carbon dioxide (effervescent decaffeination)
Alcoholic beverages	Up to 1 per day for women and people over 60 Up to 2 per day for men	Red wine Dark beer (ales and stout)
Dark chocolate	Up to 30 grams per day	Dark chocolate

CHAPTER FOURTEEN

How Soon Will You See Improvements?

When I first tried probiotics, I have to admit I was sceptical. Our laboratory research had shown that if you jumble up the gut microflora, you could cause allergic respiratory disease in mice. But creating problems is a lot easier than fixing them. And humans often respond differently from mice.

Could probiotics relieve something as tenacious as my lifelong allergies and asthma? I decided to take a probiotic supplement and to make a few simple changes in my diet, just to see what happened. Yoghurt became my new breakfast and my new bedtime snack. I also increased my intake of fruit and vegetables. Whenever possible, I substituted whole grains for processed ones. And I tried to cut back on sugar. No big deal.

Because I doubted this little experiment would work, I didn't mention it to anyone, not even my wife. And I didn't bother to record my allergy symptoms. That's why I didn't notice improvements at first. As I described in Chapter 1, my 'aha!' moment came after about a month: I'd spent the evening writing a grant proposal, a box of tissues at my side. After all these years, I knew to be prepared for the inevitable sneezing and runny nose caused by my mould allergies, which kicked up at night. But when I finished working and cleared the table, I realised that I hadn't touched the tissues. And as I looked back on the previous month, I could see other changes. This wasn't my first sneeze-free evening; I hadn't needed my asthma inhaler for several weeks. To my astonishment, the experiment had been a major success.

If you're ready to try a similar experiment of your own, you know from previous chapters how to proceed – the foods to eat, the supplements to consider. This chapter will explain what to expect as you get started, and how to make adjustments in your programme.

WHAT TO EXPECT

Doctors can practically give you a timetable when you take certain medications: 'You may feel drowsy for a couple of days, but the rash should stop itching by tomorrow and disappear by the end of the week.' We're not at that point yet with probiotics. But I'll give you a range of possibilities, based on what I know from the medical literature, as well as from my own experience and what I've heard from others. Much depends on the specific issues you're hoping to address.

Digestive Difficulties

Minor bowel problems tend to be alleviated pretty quickly. For example, if you use probiotics to counter antibiotic-associated diarrhoea, you might see a difference in just a day or two. One story I heard involved a woman who started taking probiotic supplements because she had respiratory allergies. Though that was her main concern, she also suffered from irregularity and loose stools, which made life unpredictable at times. Five days after she started the supplements, she became regular for the first time in years. The person who told me about this – someone who had never experienced irregularity – was surprised at how excited and happy this woman was about the improvement. Later, there were positive changes in her allergies, too.

If you suffer from more serious digestive problems, you should see improvements within two weeks. If not, see suggestions below on adjusting your programme.

Allergy Symptoms

My own mould allergies took several weeks to subside. In that same period, my allergic asthma improved. A more subtle change involved my food allergies. I used to develop a skin rash when I ate more than a tiny amount of beans or tomatoes. The problem didn't go away completely. But I can now eat a moderate portion of these foods. That's a good thing, because tomatoes and beans are family favourites.

Some people have told me that their allergies disappeared quickly when they started taking probiotic supplements. Others saw no effect. Will probiotics help with your allergies? As I'll describe later in this chapter, you may need to experiment with a number of foods and supplements before you'll know for sure.

Other Conditions

The same general pattern I've described for digestive and allergic conditions applies to any other problem that you hope probiotics will address. In some cases, results are seen in just a few days. But it may take up to two weeks to see improvements and then, depending on the condition, another few months to enjoy maximal relief. If you see no difference after two weeks, it's time to try something else.

Changes Over Time

Two months after I started, I had another surprise. I stepped on the scales — something I do infrequently — and discovered that I'd lost just over a stone. I couldn't believe I'd lost so much weight without trying. My first reaction was: the scales must be broken. But when I thought about it for a minute, I realised that my trousers fitted differently. There was nothing wrong with the scales.

Though I wasn't exactly overweight when I started, I had gained just over a stone since my college days. And now that excess weight was gone. I can't be sure how much of my weight loss to credit to probiotics. I had also reduced sugar and had added fruit, vegetables and whole grains to my diet. All this undoubtedly helped. If you're trying to lose weight — and you pay more attention to results than I did — you may see effects in just a week or two.

Further changes developed over time. After a medical check-up the following year — post-probiotics and post-weight loss — I learnt that my cholesterol had dropped by 20 points from 'borderline high' into the normal range. My endurance also improved. Great news for a weekend warrior who fulfils his dreams of World Cup glory by playing in an over-30 football league!

Subtle Differences

If you're taking probiotics simply to maintain good health, results will be difficult to spot. How could you know about the cold you didn't catch or the stomach upset you escaped? But after a while you may look back and realise that you've had fewer brief episodes of constipation or diarrhoea, or that you weren't felled by the twenty-four-hour bug that hit just about everyone else at work.

THE INITIAL ADJUSTMENT PERIOD

I've already mentioned that I didn't notice improvements when I first began adding probiotics. Now I'll tell you what I *did* notice: lots of intestinal wind. The problem wasn't a complete surprise. I'd read that some people experience this discomfort when first trying probiotics. It's an example of what the alternative medicine literature sometimes calls 'herx' or a 'herx reaction' – a temporary increase in symptoms on the way to recovery. 'Herx' is short for 'Jarisch-Herxheimer reaction'.

Sometimes You Get Worse Before You Get Better

More than a century ago, two European dermatologists, Adolf Jarisch and Karl Herxheimer, independently observed that when they treated patients with certain skin conditions, their symptoms actually got worse at first. In addition, the patients developed fever and nausea. These reactions continued for a few days, then were followed by improvements and healing. Why does this happen? When bacteria die, they release toxins. And the toxins can produce temporary symptoms.

Alternative medicine practitioners have taken the idea further. They use it to explain problems at the beginning of other kinds of treatment or supplement regimens. In the case of probiotics, these problems include GI tract difficulties, such as flatulence, bloating and loose stools. But some people also experience a worsening of allergic reactions or the flu-like symptoms described by Jarisch and Herxheimer.

➤ BREAKING WIND ◄

Certain bacteria in our microflora produce wind – consisting mostly of methane and hydrogen – as they digest fibre. Other types of bacteria absorb this wind, because they need it to grow. We know that our diet influences the type and amount of wind we produce. A typical Western diet favours the growth of bacteria that produce methane; people in developing countries are more likely to have a microflora that produces hydrogen. Incidentally, methane-producing bacteria are associated with inflammatory bowel disease.

Normally, the gas-producing bacteria and the gas absorbers are in sufficient balance so we don't have a lot of extra wind to expel. Nevertheless, all of us pass wind frequently, though we may not be aware of it. Usually the amounts are small; there's not necessarily any sound or smell. And sometimes it happens while we're asleep.

If you've studied chemistry, you may know that methane and hydrogen are odourless – but farts often are not. The smell comes from hydrogen sulphide and other sulphur compounds. Bacteria in our intestines create these compounds as they digest food containing sulphur. That includes eggs, meat, processed foods with sulphur compounds and various vegetables like cabbage and broccoli. Other bacteria consume the problematic sulphur compounds. The reason that some people cause more air pollution than others is that their microflora mix lacks sufficient numbers of these particular bacteria.

Though we don't yet have scientific evidence that dead bacteria in the gut are to blame, we do know that similar problems occur with antibiotic treatment, which also involves bacterial slaughter. So this explanation seems plausible to me. A new army of probiotics is now competing with the non-probiotic microbes in your digestive tract. If you began with a microflora that was out of balance, and have made significant changes in your diet and added probiotic supplements, then you've created a major microbial civil war. Microbes will be displaced or killed by the battle, leaving the microflora balance temporarily altered. The problem is exacerbated if you've also added fibre, which can have a similar effect.

Easing the Transition

The herx reactions described above are usually mild and temporary. Most people simply wait it out – that's what I did. However, if you find herx symptoms troubling, the fastest way to relieve them is to cut back on new foods and supplements. After the difficulties have subsided, start to make changes again. But this time, make them more gradually.

Another approach is to treat the symptoms. For example, if you experience a mild worsening of allergic reactions, you can get relief by taking your usual medication, such as decongestants or antihistamines.

Similarly, if the problem is wind – or associated bloating, abdominal discomfort, or loose stools – you could try an over-the-counter digestive aid. But read the label first. Anti-wind medication that contains simethicone simply changes the surface tension of gas bubbles, which allows them to leave the body more easily. That's good, because it relieves the symptoms without interfering with the adjustment process.

On the other hand, other types work differently: they contain an enzyme that breaks down the fibre in food. This reduces the amount of fibre available to the gut microbes, so they make less wind. But if they're not consuming the additional fibre you've added to your diet, the microflora won't achieve a new balance, one in which gas-consuming bacteria reach sufficient numbers to handle the amount that's normally produced. Nevertheless, if there are times during the adjustment period when intestinal wind might lead to social disaster, this type of digestive aid can save you.

If Initial Problems Don't Improve After Two Weeks

Herx reactions are normally brief. If they continue for two weeks without improvement, it's time to adjust your probiotics pro- gramme. Here are questions to ask yourself:

- **Have I increased my fibre intake too much?**
This is most likely to happen if you try to get fibre through supplements. It's easy to swallow more supplements than you really need. But it takes a lot of chewing to consume excessive fibre in the form of food. However, if you've made all the recommended changes at once – switching to whole grains, consuming the skins of fruit and vegetables – you might need to slow down temporarily.

One possibly unexpected fibre source is yoghurt. If you're eating a brand that adds fibre – look for inulin, pectin or fructo- oligosaccharides (FOS) on the label – try switching to a brand that doesn't include these ingredients, at least until your symptoms subside.

- **Am I using home-made yoghurt or kefir?**
People have made their own yoghurt and kefir for centuries. These products can be delicious and health-promoting. But you don't know exactly which types of bacteria they contain. If you're running into problems, you might have encountered a particular microbe that doesn't agree with you. Try consuming less at first or switch to a commercial version to see if that makes a difference.

- **Might I be lactose intolerant?**

If you normally don't eat dairy produce but have begun adding yoghurt, kefir or cheese to your diet, try going off them for a few days. If that solves the problem, it doesn't mean that you shouldn't try dairy foods again. Many lactose-intolerant people can eat fermented dairy products, because probiotic bacteria help to digest lactose. Try consuming smaller quantities – for example, divide a single serving into four tiny portions spread through an entire day.

- **Have I added any new food to which I might have a sensitivity or allergy?**

Eliminate that food and see if the problem goes away. This is vitally important if you experience any signs of an allergic reaction, such as hot flushes, itching or hives, swelling of your lips, vomiting or difficulty breathing.

- **Do I have any symptoms that require medical attention?**

Herx reactions aren't usually severe or alarming. Generally, they're familiar problems that come up from time to time. For example, your allergies might become a little worse than usual – but you shouldn't experience anything close to a 'worst-ever' episode. If you do, stop consuming probiotics and any new foods, and consult your GP. Be especially careful if asthma symptoms get worse. Breathing problems are always serious.

Similarly, any initial digestive problems should be minor. Discontinue what you're doing if more serious symptoms develop, such as diarrhoea that continues for more than two days; blood in the stool; digestive problems that leave you dehydrated and feeling dizzy when you stand up; and abdominal pain that isn't relieved by going to the toilet.

FINE-TUNING YOUR DIET AND SUPPLEMENTS

You may not notice changes immediately if you're taking probiotics to improve overall health. But if you were hoping for specific benefits, you can expect to see improvements after a month. If that doesn't happen, don't give up! You may need more probiotics or different ones. Some suggestions:

• If you're consuming only one or two probiotic serving units daily (see Chapter 10, pages 208–209 for details), add one more and see if that helps. Two or three units are recommended to prevent or address medical problems.

• Try a different mix of probiotic foods so that you're consuming different microbes. For example, if your yoghurt contains only the standard starter cultures – *Lactobacillus bulgaricus* and *Streptococcus thermophilus* – see if you get better results from a brand that has additional bacteria. Or broaden your horizons (and probiotic consumption) with kefir.

• Increase your consumption of prebiotics, within the nutrition guidelines suggested in Chapter 13. Try a yoghurt that contains added prebiotics – inulin, pectin or fructo-oligosaccharides (FOS).

• Add a probiotic supplement, using the advice in Chapter 11.

• If you're already taking a probiotic supplement, use the guidelines in Chapter 11 to determine if a larger dose would be appropriate. Remember that not all probiotic microbes are equally effective against all health problems. Consider switching to another supplement that contains a different mix of probiotics, or adding a supplement that supplies a new type.

• If you're not getting results from a supplement that isn't on the list of recommended brands in Chapter 11, try a brand that's on the list. Though the list isn't complete and undoubtedly omits many good products, we know from consumer studies that some supplements don't contain what's promised on the label.

THE ONGOING ADJUSTMENT PROCESS

Your microflora is a living community of microbes. Changes in your life can affect the healthy balance you've achieved. Moving to a different location may mean different microbes in your food and water. Marriage or a change in your job may affect your diet. Your level of emotional stress can go up or down. And physical changes – including illness, pregnancy and weight loss – can alter your microflora. If the probiotics programme that worked before no longer has the same beneficial effects, it's time to retune.

If You Become Pregnant

Follow the nutritional guidelines you receive from your antenatal healthcare provider, but try to make choices within those guidelines to favour probiotics and prebiotics. If you've been using a probiotic supplement, ask if it's okay to continue. And you might want to reread Chapter 5, which describes research showing benefits to expectant mums and their babies.

If You Experience Acute Diarrhoea

Acute diarrhoea can result from antibiotic use, a stomach virus, food poisoning or other illnesses. Think of it as a tornado ripping through your GI tract, sweeping away many of the microbes that normally live there. Your microflora may be temporarily unbalanced after you recover, so you may experience digestive problems for a while. See if you can tolerate additional probiotics during this period, because they may help. If the problem persists, talk to your GP.

If You Need to Take Medication

Some people (and, unfortunately, some doctors) take a 'don't ask; don't tell' position on supplements. That's not a good idea. Just as your healthcare providers need to know what prescription and over-the-counter medications you use, they should know about your probiotic consumption.

Certain medications affect the microflora, directly or indirectly. The table on the next page explains how to make sure your medication and probiotics work effectively together.

This chapter has focused on the early stage of taking probiotics – a period when you'll probably be paying more attention than usual to your diet and to your physical well-being. I hope it doesn't sound as if adding probiotics is like taking on a second job. Because it's not! I'm sure that, like me, you'll soon find that probiotics are part of your life.

Today, our kitchen is stocked with yoghurt and kefir, just as the bathroom cupboard is stocked with toothpaste. When I travel and can't follow my usual diet, I automatically use supplements to make up for what I'm missing. But what I will never take for granted are all the improvements I've gained from probiotics. All it takes is a glorious summer day to remind me that I can now take a deep breath and enjoy the fragrant air, without having to worry about pollen triggering an allergic reaction.

HELPING MEDICATION AND PROBIOTICS WORK TOGETHER
(Adjust probiotic foods and supplements as indicated.)

TYPE OF DRUG	WHAT'S THE ISSUE?	WHAT TO DO
Antibiotic	Kills probiotic bacteria, such as *Lactobacillus* and *Bifidobacterium,* as well as targeted bacteria. Note: probiotic yeasts, such as *Saccharomyces boulardii,* are not affected by antibiotics.	Consume probiotic bacteria at least two hours after taking antibiotics. A probiotic yeast can be taken at the same time as antibiotics.
Systemic oral antifungal medications (e.g. fluconazole, nystatin)	Kills probiotic yeast, such as *Saccharomyces boulardii,* as well as harmful yeasts. Note: probiotic bacteria, such as *Lactobacillus* and *Bifidobacterium,* are not affected by antifungal medications.	Take probiotic yeast at least two hours after taking antifungal drugs. Probiotic bacteria can be consumed at the same time as antifungals.
Antacids and acid blockers, such as Tagamet	Counters desirable presence of acid in the stomach and the beginning of the small intestine; acid controls growth of harmful bacteria, creating a selective advantage for probiotic bacteria.	If you must take any of these medications, increase the dose or frequency of probiotics. Gradually work up to double the usual amount of probiotics for as long as the medication is needed.
Non-steroidal anti-inflammatory drugs, such as aspirin	Can block production of stomach acid; this acid normally gives probiotic bacteria a competitive advantage.	
Laxatives and any drug that lists diarrhoea as a side effect	Speeds emptying of intestinal contents, including probiotic bacteria.	
Muscle relaxants or any drug that lists constipation as a side effect	Decreases peristalsis, which slows emptying of intestinal contents, allowing competing bacteria to proliferate.	

CHAPTER FIFTEEN

Making Probiotics a Family Affair

Long before I started my personal experiment with probiotics, my wife and I had begun to see signs of allergic reactions in our children. At the age of 4, our daughter developed eczema after eating peanut butter – a food we immediately removed from her diet. A few years later, she became short of breath while playing football, raising concerns about exercise-induced asthma. We had also noticed that our son, then a toddler, developed eczema on his feet after he wore certain shoes. This led to much experimentation with different types of footwear.

We knew that allergies tend to run in families. You can imagine how distressed I was by these signs that my children might be destined to share the problem that had plagued my life. But with the success of my experiment came the hope that we could head it off.

Healthy eating was already a concern for my wife and me. Our diet reflected that – well, at least most of the time. We had been working on getting the kids to eat more fruit, vegetables and whole grains – in other words, we had unknowingly tried to increase their intake of prebiotics. Now we wanted to go much further. We knew it would be a challenge. Neither of us had hours to spend on shopping and food preparation. Our personal probiotics revolution had to be efficient to succeed. In addition to making our new diet compatible with our busy lives, we needed to make it palatable to the children. Our son was 7 at that point; our daughter was 10. Clearly, a variety of strategies would be required to encourage them to cooperate.

PROBIOTIC SURVIVAL TIPS FOR SUPER-BUSY PEOPLE

I understand what it's like to deal with hectic mornings, a demanding job with short lunch breaks (if I'm lucky), complicated school run schedules and days that leave little time to make dinner. My wife is just as busy as I am. Labourious food preparation is not an option. Of necessity, we've learnt to be efficient. Fortunately, it's not all that complicated or time-consuming to follow the guidelines in this book. I'll share some of our tips below.

Probiotics and Prebiotics Are Fast Foods, Too

Here are a few of my family's favourite foods for those times when meals must be 'grab and run'. Each is ready to eat in less than thirty seconds. Just put an assortment on the table and let everyone help themselves. My children think it's cool to have breakfast cereal for dinner. Of course, it's a low-sugar prebiotic-rich cereal with fruit on top (or on the side, if they prefer).

- Yoghurt
- Aged cheese
- Peanut butter
- Hummus
- Muesli and other high-fibre cereals (preferably low in sugar and fat)
- Whole grain bread
- Whole grain crackers (preferably low salt)
- Ready-to-eat vegetables: baby carrots, celery slices, pepper strips
- Berries, grapes, cherries
- Whole fruit, such as an orange, apple, or banana
- Dried fruit (preferably unsweetened)
- Trail mix
- Nuts

Manufacturers are wising up. These days, it's almost as easy to buy a one-serving bag of baby carrots to tuck into a lunch box as it is to buy a bag of crisps. Next time you're in a supermarket or health food store, take a few extra minutes to explore. Among the 'convenient but healthy' options I've discovered are single-serving bags of salads, dried fruit, trail mix and baked whole grain snacks. For a quick hot breakfast or lunch, look for cups that contain instant whole grain cereal or high-fibre bean soup – just add boiling water and stir. You don't even have to wash up.

Time Shifting

We take the pressure off weekday rush hours at breakfast and dinner by shifting food preparation chores to evenings or weekends.

- Blend fruit (frozen berries are great) and yoghurt in the evening, store in the refrigerator – and have an instant smoothie the following morning.
- Over the weekend, create your own salad bar for the week. Wash and cut up vegetables – peppers, celery, carrots, cucumbers, broccoli, red onions – and store them in bags or containers in the refrigerator. As I'll describe later in this chapter, I often make a supply of grated carrots for the week. You can also prepare vegetables – as assistants do for professional chefs – to streamline stir-fries, steaming or baking. Just store them sealed in the refrigerator. For example: wash and cut up fresh broccoli and cauliflower on Sunday for a quick stir-fry on Wednesday.
- Cut up cheese ahead of time and store in containers in the fridge.
- Use the weekend to cook foods that require simmering or baking time but little effort or attention, such as soups, sauces, stews, beans, brown rice or baked sweet potato. Soups, sauces and stews actually pick up flavour as they sit in the fridge.

A Quick Sprinkling of Prebiotics

Herbs and spices are loaded with dietary phenols, which are valuable prebiotics. To make it easy to add them to food, we keep containers of our favourite herbs on the table – oregano, basil, Italian seasoning mix and onion powder – along with the salt and pepper. I love the flavour of oregano and routinely sprinkle it on sandwich fillings, soups, salads and grilled meat or poultry. Your family might prefer a different mix, such as one involving hot pepper, cumin and curry powder.

Substitutions

Look for substitution opportunities that add probiotics and pre-biotics to your favourite recipes. Using more healthy ingredients doesn't take any longer. Sometimes you'll need to tinker a bit to come up with the best formula. And you may want to introduce certain changes gradually so your family can get accustomed to the new version.

HEALTHY FOOD SWAPS
TO ADD PROBIOTICS AND PREBIOTICS

INSTEAD OF	USE
Regular white bread and pasta	Wholewheat or whole grain versions
White flour for baking	All or part wholewheat flour
White flour or cornstarch for thickening sauces and stews	Finely chopped or grated vegetables, mashed or chopped beans such as refried beans, ground flaxseed, oat bran, wheatgerm or wheat bran
White flour or white breadcrumbs for coating chicken or fish	Whole grain breadcrumbs, oatmeal or oat bran
Butter, margarine and other less healthy fats for cooking	Olive oil, peanut oil and other healthier fats
Butter, margarine and other less healthy fats for baking	Rapeseed oil, soya bean oil and other healthier fats
Mayonnaise or soured cream in dips or dressings	Start by using yoghurt for a third of the mayonnaise or soured cream; gradually increase the proportion of yoghurt
Milk or cream in baking	Substitute yoghurt for all or part; add ½ teaspoon of baking soda for each measure of yoghurt
Soured cream or buttermilk in baking	Substitute yoghurt for all or part

HOW DO I GET MY KIDS TO EAT THIS STUFF?

If your children favour the kinds of foods that most children do, getting them to eat plain yoghurt, wholewheat pasta and apples with the skin on may seem impossible. But we've found that a gradual approach is surprisingly effective and painless. This involves slow introduction of new foods (sometimes in sneaky ways) along with efforts at persuasion. I bet this approach would work with sceptical adults, too.

I don't want to imply that junk food never enters our home or that everything we eat would pass muster with the Nutrition Police. Nor would I urge such perfection on anyone else. However, occasional lapses aren't a serious problem – provided that you consume probiotics and prebiotics most of the time.

The 'One Bite' Rule

We've always encouraged our children to try new foods. Our long-standing rule is that they must take one small taste – about a tablespoon – of whatever is being served. If they don't like it, they don't have to eat any more. And to avoid insulting the chef, especially when they eat away from home, we trained them years ago to say 'Thank you, but I don't care for this' if they encounter a food they dislike. I know the phrase sounds a bit formal coming from a child, but it sure beats 'Eeewww – that's *disgusting*!'

I remember the evening my wife decided to introduce whole-wheat pasta for the first time. She's a terrific cook and enjoys trying new recipes. She had found a pasta recipe that involved asparagus, garlic, olive oil, thyme, rosemary and grated parmesan. Because the dish sounded so delicious, she had made a special trip to the store to buy fresh asparagus and herbs earlier that day.

Our son put the required forkful in his mouth. A pained expression came over his face and he didn't swallow. His lips were pressed together and his cheeks were puffed out. He looked so

➤➤ RESEARCH SUPPORT FOR THE 'ONE BITE' RULE ➤➤

Many youngsters resist trying new foods – especially vegetables. Psychologists refer to this phenomenon as 'food neophobia'. Neophobia is a fear of anything new. (Mysteriously, the problem doesn't come up with puddings.) Experimental evidence confirms what many parents have discovered on their own: the most effective way to get past food neophobia is to repeatedly expose the child to the food until it becomes more familiar. Exposure doesn't mean forcing a child to eat a whole portion of aubergine. Repeated tiny tastes do the trick. And – this may be surprising – mere exposure works better than bribery.

Researchers from University College in London randomly assigned 49 children aged 5 to 7 to one of three groups to see if they could encourage a taste for raw sweet red pepper. Over a two-week period, children in one group were offered a minor bribe (a cartoon sticker) if they'd eat at least one piece of pepper; those in the other group were simply asked to taste the pepper. Both groups were invited to eat as much additional pepper as they wished. The third group, the controls, weren't given this extra exposure to the peppers.

After eight days, the two groups of children who had been offered the peppers were significantly more likely than the control group to eat them willingly. In fact, some of these children now thought the peppers were delicious. But the children who liked them the most were the ones who were just asked to take a taste. Those who were bribed were not quite as enthusiastic. The study was published in the *European Journal of Clinical Nutrition* in 2003.

distressed that I feared he was having an allergic reaction. He grabbed his glass of water and gulped it, washing down the pasta and asparagus. Then he gasped, 'Thank you, but I don't care for this.'

Over time, experimentation has become easier. Our children now have a sense of adventure about food. To be honest, some of the things we've tasted were not very good – even 'horrible', according to our children. But we've had lots of successes, too. And when we cashed in our frequent-flier miles and took the children to Germany and France during a school holiday, I was amazed at how willingly they tried sauerkraut, exotic sausages, unfamiliar yoghurts and the stinkiest of cheeses.

Cutting Back on Sugar

Our kids, like most, love sweets. One of our goals when we changed the family's diet was to cut back drastically on sugar. Replacing it with artificial sweeteners wasn't an attractive option as far as we were concerned. Even if sweeteners have no calories, they contribute to an appetite for sweets. And we can't be certain that they're risk-free. We never planned to eliminate sugar altogether. Rather, our goal was to gradually reduce how much we were eating by becoming more selective about sweets and by getting accustomed to less sweetness in our food.

The Yoghurt Transition

Yoghurt was already a staple in our house when we began our new eating programme – but all of us ate sweetened versions. At the time, our refrigerator was stocked with two kinds: grown-up yoghurt that contained fruit preserves, and kids' yoghurt that tasted like pudding. It came in a container decorated with animal characters; an attached packet provided crumbled biscuits to sprinkle on the yoghurt to make it even sweeter.

➤➤ TEACHING AN OLD DOG A NEW TRICK ➤➤

We have two dogs. Murphy, who's 10 years old, is a golden retriever. He has what vets call 'old dog lungs'. About six months ago, we noticed that he seemed short of breath and was coughing. Dogs don't normally cough, so we took him to the vet. She prescribed a strong broad-spectrum antibiotic, in case he had a bacterial infection. If that didn't work, we could try an antihistamine. She warned us that Murphy probably would get diarrhoea when he was on the antibiotic.

My wife and I talked about what to do. I suggested plain yoghurt. 'He's a dog,' I said. 'He'll eat anything.' My wife was sceptical; she wondered if he'd like the tart taste. But what could we lose by trying? We put about half a cup of plain yoghurt in a bowl and held it out to Murphy. He began lapping it up.

The sound caught the attention of our younger dog, Duke, a Labrador retriever. Murphy was eating something that he wasn't getting! Duke raced into the kitchen and tried to stick his nose in the bowl. We quickly gave him his own dish of yoghurt.

Murphy got through the course of antibiotics without diarrhoea. The drug didn't help, but his symptoms improved on the antihistamine. So we presume he has allergies. When we told the vet about feeding Murphy yoghurt to prevent diarrhoea, she thought that was a good idea. She'd been using probiotics to treat a cat with symptoms of chronic kidney disease – a common problem in older cats – and had been amazed at the improvement.

We still try to give Murphy and Duke a heaped spoonful of yoghurt daily. Both dogs come running when they hear the sound of a yoghurt container opening. At this point, Murphy no longer needs antihistamines. He rarely coughs and his shortness of breath is much better.

When our supply of kids' yoghurt ran out, we didn't replace it. Instead, we gave the children our yoghurt. They reacted as if we'd presented them with spoilt food: 'This is *sour!*' We compromised by letting them crush a few biscuits and mix them in. But over time, they became accustomed to tarter yoghurt and gave up the biscuits. Meanwhile, I made the transition to plain yoghurt by mixing decreasing amounts of sweetened yoghurt into it. Sometimes, if the children aren't paying attention, I can get away with giving them a mixture that's half sweetened and half plain.

The Sugar Budget

To become more sugar-aware, we put the children (and ourselves) on a sugar budget. We allow them to decide how to 'spend' their sugar allocation each day. For example, we let them choose between drinking a fizzy drink with dinner or having pudding – the budget doesn't allow for both. We encourage them to enjoy whichever treat they've selected.

I've already mentioned our transition to yoghurt that's less sweet. If you prefer sweetened yoghurt, no problem. Just apply the sugar budget idea: cut out a can of fizzy drink or a few biscuits to compensate. Thanks to the probiotics in the yoghurt, you'll come out ahead. Here are other measures we've used to tame the family sweet tooth:

• **Turn sugary cereals into cereal toppings.** As with yoghurt, we made the transition from sugary cereals to low-sugar cereals by mixing the two. Over time, we cut back on the amount of sugary cereal. At this point, a thin layer on top of a serving of low-sugar cereal is enough to satisfy the children's morning sugar craving.

• **Include fruit with dessert.** A small scoop of ice cream or a narrow slice of cake looks more lavish if it's heaped with a generous portion of berries or cut-up fruit.

- **Redefine fizzy drinks as a treat rather than a thirst-quenching beverage.** My children still drink fizzy drinks occasionally, but as a treat. When they're simply thirsty, they drink water.

Because we made changes gradually, cutting sugar consumption was less of a challenge than I'd expected. As we reduced the amount of sugar we ate, our appetite for sweets shrank, too. Interestingly, both kids began to notice that if they ate a lot of sugary food, they didn't feel very well.

➤ 'I'M NOT GOING TO EAT THE SKIN!' ⭠

Because fruit and vegetable skins contain phenols, they're bitter. And to make matters worse, the skin also changes the texture. So it's not surprising that kids don't like unpeeled fruit and vegetables at first. Before we began our new eating programme, my wife and I peeled off fruit and vegetable skins upon request. But now we were reluctant to take off the very part that contained most of the valuable dietary phenols and fibre.

Our children always loved apples. But simply handing them an unpeeled apple didn't work in the beginning. Nor did they find big chunks of unpeeled apples acceptable – a chunk still required chewing through a lot of skin. Finally, we cut an unpeeled apple into really thin slices. That worked. With thin slices, there was plenty of the sweet apple centre and just a sliver of skin. By the way, even though I'm a middle-aged adult, this is my favourite way to eat an apple.

I want to emphasise that our house is not a sugar-free zone. All of us still enjoy puddings. But we no longer want gargantuan portions. Sugar-loaded foods have moved from staples of the children's daily diet to infrequent treats. When the kids have friends over for a party or sleepover, we set out fizzy drinks and provide sweet snacks. But these special occasions are just that – special and occasional.

Let's Make a Deal

Our family has a long tradition of eating waffles for breakfast at the weekend. One week we bought frozen wholewheat waffles instead of our usual buttermilk waffles. The kids took the required taste and responded: 'Thank you, but I don't care for this.'

We didn't insist that they eat the waffles, but this wasn't the end of it. One Sunday, just before the kids came downstairs for breakfast, I made the wholewheat waffles again. My daughter loves fruit. So I left her waffles plain but prepared a big bowl of strawberry purée by emptying a packet of frozen strawberries (with no sugar added) into a bowl and mashing them. For my son, I put a couple of tablespoons of chocolate chips on each waffle, and then stuck them in the microwave briefly to melt the chocolate chips. We'd always set limits on the amount of syrup they could use, but the syrup bottle was nowhere in sight for this experiment.

I told my daughter, 'Take as much strawberry sauce as you'd like.' She buried the waffles under a pile of strawberry purée and dug in. The chocolate chips won over my son. This breakfast provided more whole grains and dietary phenols than the old version – and actually had slightly less sugar. The perfect compromise.

⚓ IT'S ALL IN THE PRESENTATION ⚓

This is an idea borrowed from the great chefs of Europe: make food look attractive. Needless to say, I don't have hours to spend on carving radish roses. But here are a few quick tricks to give health-promoting foods extra visual appeal:

• Layer yoghurt and berries in a parfait glass or other clear glass.

• Add sprinkles. A teaspoon of colored sprinkles adds minimal sugar, but it helped convince our son to eat a more tart-tasting yoghurt than his previous favourite.

• Make whole grain pancakes with initials: dribble batter onto the grill to form an initial, written backwards. Allow it to cook for half a minute. Then pour batter over it to make a pancake. When you flip the pancake, the initial, which has cooked longer, will be darker than the rest.

• Use biscuit cutters to make slices of cheese into hearts and other interesting shapes.

• Slice carrots into 'golden coins'.

• Buy fruit and vegetables in new colours. Our kids enjoy pepper slices in yellow and orange, as well as the usual green and red.

• Arrange carrots, celery and other cut-up vegetables on a plate and put a small bowl of dip or dressing in the middle. Peanut butter is also a great topper for sliced celery, apples and bananas.

• Use novelty dishes – for example, colourful souvenir plates or cups – just for certain healthy foods.

Hide the Prebiotics

Children may reject new foods simply because they 'look funny'. We've worked out ways to hide prebiotics in familiar foods. My favourite hiding place is pasta sauce. (See Chapter 16 for the recipe.) The strong tomato flavour masks quite a few secret ingredients, selected for their nutritional power. I thicken the sauce with ground carrots (ground, not grated, chopped or sliced, which yields a different texture) or a tablespoon or two of refried beans, bran or ground flaxseed – all of which contain valuable prebiotics, including fibre. Since tomato is acidic, I sweeten the sauce slightly with a small amount of prebiotic-rich juice: Concord grape, pomegranate or whatever other dark berry juice I have on hand.

Because the flavour of this pasta sauce is so rich, I don't get objections when I serve it with wholewheat pasta. I top the sauce with grated cheese and oregano. My equivalent of a three-star rating came from one of my son's friends who observed, 'This tastes just like a pizza. Can I have more?'

The sauce is known as 'Dad's Secret Recipe', because I've never revealed ingredients such as bran or refried beans, which might provoke comments like 'That's *nasty*!' The sauce goes into other Italian dishes, such as lasagne or quick pizzas made with slices of whole grain bread and grated cheese – and I occasionally serve it over leftover brown rice as a side dish. I use the same basic technique to add hidden prebiotics to chilli, vegetable soup and other casseroles.

Here are some of our other 'hide the prebiotic' tricks:

• Oregano is one of the most potent prebiotics, but we all know how most children feel about green flakes in their food. We mix oregano into one of the children's favourites: ketchup. Since they love pizza, and this looks like pizza sauce – a trustworthy food – they've never objected to the green specks.

• At the weekend, we grind about two pounds of scrubbed,

unpeeled carrots in the food processor. We store the carrots – which look like orange minced meat – in a container in the refrigerator. During the week, we use them to top salads, tacos and cheese-stuffed pitta bread. We also put them into soups and sauces and into meat destined to become tacos or burgers. Somehow, they're not as noticeable as grated or chopped carrots, especially in a tomato-based sauce or soup. But they add a slight sweetness and crunch that my children really like.

• Tinned refried beans, which are loaded with fibre, make an excellent thickener and flavouring for just about any sauce or gravy that goes with a beefy flavour. Despite the reference to frying in the name, many brands are low in fat – just check the label. They're already mashed and couldn't be more convenient. Be warned: if you add too much, the sauce will become pasty. However, a heaped spoonful or two works well in many recipes.

• Add ground flaxseed – which is rich in fibre and omega-3 fatty acids – to thicken soups, gravies, tomato sauce, pancakes, muffins and other baked goods.

Getting Hunger on Our Side

Everyone has a big appetite just before dinner, so we take advantage of that. We put slices of raw veggies or fruit into a bowl and invite the children to help themselves while we prepare the rest of the meal. Sometimes I slice apples and make a ring around a plate, with baby carrots in the centre. This looks good.

Dinner often starts with salad. We've found that our kids are more willing to eat it at the beginning of the meal, because that's when they're hungriest. They eat the salad even faster if the main course is something they really like. This trick has helped them accept the more bitter nutrient-rich dark greens we now serve instead of iceberg lettuce.

If we're having pudding, we usually delay it for about half an hour. That way, the kids are no longer hungry. They still want the sweet flavour, but that desire is satisfied with a much smaller portion.

Pushing Healthy Snacks and Drinks

When kids have friends over to play, they'll grab whatever is readily available. So we stock the refrigerator and worktops with items like fresh whole fruit, dried fruit, berries, grapes, whole grain snack bars and veggie strips with a dip. You've heard the expression 'out of sight, out of mind' – this is 'in sight, in mind'. We've been amazed at how often kids grab a carrot, apple slice or celery stick as they walk past the counter during the day.

As I mentioned earlier, we encourage our children to quench their thirst with water. One trick that works is to fill small bottles with water and store them in the refrigerator. When they're thirsty, our kids can grab a cold bottle of water. My son has remarked, 'These are really refreshing!'

We also keep a supply of healthy drinks on hand, such as milk, orange juice and phenol-rich dark juices, like pomegranate or blueberry. These are usually mixed with tonic water – our standard ratio is one part juice to four parts of tonic water – and served over ice. This is also an excellent non-alcoholic 'cocktail' for adult parties.

Friendly Persuasion

Most parents step up to the podium every once in a while and deliver a lecture on the importance of healthy eating. We can't help ourselves. But it's impossible not to notice – especially if kids roll their eyes and mutter 'Bor-ring' – that lectures aren't the best way to get the message across. Here are two techniques that my wife and I have found more effective. Maybe they'll work for your family, too.

➤ INVOLVING KIDS IN FOOD PREPARATION ➤

One of the most effective ways to change children's eating habits is to involve them in food preparation. A few suggestions:

• When they grow it, they will eat it. My daughter tends the small garden on the side of our house where we grow tomatoes, red and green peppers, courgettes, basil and oregano. If you don't have a garden, you can cultivate a few vegetables in pots placed on a windowsill. Even a tiny harvest – say, a handful of runner beans – makes that vegetable more acceptable.

• Let children participate in shopping decisions. Have each child select one new fruit or vegetable to try each week. That's how we discovered yellow and orange peppers.

• Encourage children to help with food preparation. Depending on their age and skills, they could research new recipes, wash and pick over berries, cut up tomatoes – or take over the kitchen and make dinner.

Our son made his first dinner for the family when he was 11. His class was working on reports about different states, and he'd selected Texas. So he decided to make chilli. Though this wasn't a food he'd liked before, he researched recipes and made up a shopping list. My wife took him to the supermarket and let him pick out all the ingredients. He prepared the chilli, tasting as he went. We all liked it. He was very proud of himself, and now he enjoys tasting other chilli recipes when we go out to eat.

Bring in Other Authorities

We save newspaper and magazine articles about healthy eating, then show the articles to our children and discuss them. This lets them know that their parents aren't the only ones recommending this food.

Make It Personal

Whenever possible, we take the opportunity to provide personal examples – involving people the children know – that show the positive effects of good nutrition. My kids know all about my life-long allergies; they've seen the recent dramatic improvements for themselves. They also know that they're at risk for allergies, and they take that very seriously. One of my son's friends can't play in our house because we have pets and he has allergies. His eyes water and he begins to sneeze if he comes inside. Our children love animals, and they don't want to lose the ability to spend time with their pets.

Though I'll never know what would have happened if we hadn't introduced probiotics and prebiotics, I do know that neither of my children suffers from allergies now. Our son is eczema-free, regardless of what shoes he wears. My daughter has no signs of asthma or any other respiratory allergies. We cautiously reintro-duced her to peanut butter, and she happily eats peanut butter sandwiches with no problem.

Our gradual transition to a healthier family diet is an ongoing journey. But as I worked on this chapter, I realised that we've come a long way. It was the end of summer and my wife took the children to Chicago for a few days to visit her family and college friends – a trip they've made many times. I stayed at home to write.

The drive to Chicago takes about four hours, so they always take plenty of snacks. Five years ago that would have meant crisps, biscuits, sweets and crackers. This year, the snack bag included single-serving yoghurts, fruit, carrots, pepper strips, trail mix, cheese and cereal bars. After they left, I went to the refrigerator to get something to eat – and discovered they'd taken all the apples!

CHAPTER SIXTEEN

Recipes

Over the past few years, as my family changed our way of eating, our way of cooking changed, too. My wife and I modified our old standbys to boost probiotic and prebiotic content; we also came up with new recipes. In this chapter, I share a few family favourites – dishes that are not just healthy, but also easy to prepare, with ample taste appeal for both children and grown-ups.

In addition to trying new recipes, I hope you'll be on the lookout for enjoyable ways to add probiotics and prebiotics to your food – stirring a spoonful of yoghurt into a cup of soup, tucking a forkful of sauerkraut into a sandwich, sprinkling fresh or dried herbs on a salad. In most cases we don't know the exact probiotic or prebiotic content of these extras, and quantities are small. But it all adds up to a healthier (and often more flavoursome) diet.

BREAKFAST

MUESLI AND YOGHURT WITH FRESH FRUIT

I am not a morning person, but I look forward to starting my day with a cup of dark-roasted coffee and a bowl of muesli, yoghurt and fruit. I also enjoy this combination as a snack, quick dinner or night-time hunger-buster.

For 1 serving:

110 grams muesli
180 ml plain or vanilla low-fat yoghurt, or a combination
110 grams fresh fruit (blueberries, raspberries, sliced strawberries, diced, unpeeled apples or peaches or other fruit)

Place muesli in a bowl, add yoghurt and top with fresh fruit. Or serve in a parfait glass and create an eye-appealing six-layer pudding: use half the muesli, yoghurt and fruit to make the first three layers; then create three more layers with the remaining muesli, yoghurt and fruit.

Notes: Try to select a muesli that's low in sugar (10 grams or less per serving). Look for prebiotic-rich ingredients, such as pumpkin seeds, nuts and flaxseed. Whole grain cereal or uncooked rolled oats can be used instead of muesli. Rolled oats have a slightly sweet taste and a chewy consistency.

If fresh fruit is not in season, use unsweetened frozen fruit such as raspberries (my personal favourite), blueberries or strawberries. Or substitute 55 grams of dried fruit such as raisins, cherries or blueberries. This is a convenient option if you're travelling.

TOASTED SOURDOUGH BREAD WITH BERRY FRUIT SPREAD

When I was a kid, my parents always told me not to spread too much jam on my toast. However, if I'm using a berry spread made with puréed fruit and no added sugar, I can load up my toast and feel like a kid sneaking extras. The sweetness of the fruit spread complements the tartness of the sourdough bread.

For 1 serving:

2 slices whole grain sourdough bread
60 grams spread made with puréed berries (blueberry, raspberry, strawberry, mixed berry)

Toast the bread. Top with the berry spread – which is full of dietary phenols – and enjoy.

Note: Check the labels and look for a berry spread that contains less than 9 grams of sugar per tablespoon of spread. There are excellent-tasting options with just 5 to 8 grams of sugar per tablespoon.

FRUIT YOGHURT SMOOTHIES

These are the powerhouses of quick breakfast drinks, loaded with phenols from the fruit, plus probiotics from the yoghurt. You can make them the night before, store them in the refrigerator – then just pour the next morning. But don't limit smoothies to breakfast. They also make a terrific snack or pudding, especially if you love milkshakes.

For 3 servings, each approximately 240 ml:

230 grams sliced fresh or frozen unsweetened strawberries
1 banana, peeled and sliced
120 ml orange juice
240 ml plain or vanilla low-fat yoghurt, or a combination
1 teaspoon vanilla extract

Place all ingredients in a blender and blend until smooth.

Notes: Instead of strawberries, substitute other fresh or frozen berries (for example, blueberries or raspberries), or diced fruit such as mango or peaches. You can also substitute 110 grams of other fruit for the banana.

Be aware that the fruit smoothies you buy in stores usually aren't made with yoghurt and often have a high sugar content. Sometimes they're prepared with ice, fruit-flavoured syrup and a banana. They may taste good, but don't fool yourself into thinking they're a health food.

SANDWICHES

REUBEN SANDWICH

Though this popular sandwich was invented in the United States, I consider the ingredients a tribute to my ethnic German heritage. If prepared with fresh sauerkraut and authentic pumpernickel bread, a Reuben sandwich is rich in probiotics and prebiotics, as well as flavour.

For 1 sandwich:

2 slices whole grain pumpernickel bread
1 tablespoon Thousand Island Yoghurt Dressing (see page 355)
60 grams fresh sauerkraut, drained
85 grams corned beef, sliced
30 grams Swiss cheese, sliced
Pinch of caraway seeds
Fermented gherkin (optional garnish)

Spread the dressing on both slices of the bread. On one slice, place sauerkraut, corned beef and cheese. Sprinkle with caraway seeds. Top with the other slice of bread. Garnish sandwich with a fermented gherkin if desired.

Notes: To maximise the probiotic value of this sandwich, use the fresh sauerkraut that's sold in refrigerated sections. Tinned sauerkraut has been heated during processing, which destroys the lactic acid bacteria.

Use high-quality pumpernickel bread. Rye flour should be the first ingredient, listed before wheat flour, if wheat flour is listed at all. In the best of all worlds, it will also be a sourdough bread, but this is hard to find. Traditionally, pumpernickel was a slow-baked sourdough bread made from rye flour and rye meal, with no wheat. The loaves were dense, dark and coarse, and noted for their strong flavour. Unfortunately, modern pumpernickel bread rarely follows this recipe. Wheat flour is usually the main ingredient, standard bread yeast supplies the leavening and the dark colour is created by adding molasses or cocoa. The resulting pumpernickel is lighter in texture and less flavoursome.

You can substitute whole grain sourdough or rye bread for the pumpernickel. Other variations: substitute pastrami or turkey for corned beef; these versions are sometimes called a Rachel sandwich. Or make a vegetarian version by omitting the meat and using smoked Gouda cheese. If you don't have Thousand Island dressing, use stone-ground brown mustard instead. Reuben sandwiches are often grilled, but that might destroy the probiotics. So I prefer them this way.

A SANDWICH MAKEOVER FOR THE PROBIOTIC REVOLUTION

Enhance your favourite sandwiches with probiotics and prebiotics, making them more flavourful as well as more nutritious. Add extra phenols by serving with iced tea.

ENHANCERS	BECAUSE
Whole grain or sourdough bread	Whole grain breads contain soluble fibre, a prebiotic. Sourdough breads contain metabiotics, the beneficial metabolic by-products of probiotic bacteria.
Mustard or dressing (see recipes on pages 354–356 for Yoghurt Ranch Dressing or Thousand Island Yoghurt Dressing)	Mustard is an antimicrobial, which can have prebiotic effects. Yoghurt (contained in some dressings) is a probiotic if dressing is prepared without heat.

Extras:
    Aged fermented cheese, such as Swiss, cheddar or Gouda
    Bean spread, such as hummus
	Aged cheese contains probiotics.
	
	Beans contain dietary phenols and soluble fibre, both prebiotics.

Vegetable toppings, such as lettuce, tomato slices, onion slices, pepper strips, ground carrots	Contain dietary phenols, which are antioxidants and prebiotics.
A dash of herbs, such as oregano or basil	Herbs and spices are a rich source of dietary phenols.

Accompaniments, such as
    Fermented gherkins
    Fresh sauerkraut
    Sliced apples or other fresh fruit
	Contain probiotics.
	Source of probiotics, metabiotics and fibre.
	Contain dietary phenols and fibre, which are prebiotics.

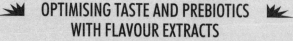 OPTIMISING TASTE AND PREBIOTICS WITH FLAVOUR EXTRACTS

Take advantage of cooking chemistry to get the most flavour – and nutrition – from herbs, spices, garlic and onion. This technique also can cut down on cooking time, because long simmering isn't needed to extract the flavour of herbs and spices.

Dietary phenols don't dissolve well in water at room temperature. Boiling liquid extracts the phenols from herbs and spices – but prolonged exposure to high temperature reduces the phenol content. That's what happens when you follow typical recipes for soups or stews, which simmer for hours. A better approach is to create a flavour extract with a small amount of wine and olive oil; phenols readily dissolve in wine or oil. Then add the extract as a finishing touch when cooking is complete.

Preparing a flavour extract is as easy as making salad dressing. Start with whatever herbs and spices your recipe calls for; you can also include garlic or onion. Add a small amount of wine (preferably red wine to maximise dietary phenol content). Typically 60 ml of wine is about right, but the exact amount doesn't matter. Combine in a blender or shake in a jar with a secure lid. Allow the mixture to sit briefly while you prepare the dish. The alcohol in the wine will begin to dissolve some of the phenols in the herbs. After a few minutes, add about 2 tablespoons of olive oil to the extract and blend again; here, too, you could use more or less.

Add the flavour extract to a soup, sauce, stew or casserole after it's stopped simmering. Using wine as well as oil will help the extract to blend in. The small amount of alcohol will evaporate when the extract is added to the hot dish.

The flavour extract can be prepared in advance. Cover, and let it stand at room temperature for up to four hours. Or make it the day before and store it in the refrigerator. It can even be frozen.

The following recipe makes enough flavour extract for 10 typical family-sized recipes. Freeze it and use as needed. This is a great way to store extra herbs from a herb garden or farmers' market at the end of summer, so you can enjoy their fresh flavours all year.

15 garlic cloves (or more or less, depending on how much you like garlic)
230 grams chopped fresh herbs such as oregano, basil or thyme (or 80 grams dried herbs)
310 ml red wine
160 ml extra virgin olive oil

Blend the garlic, herbs, wine and olive oil together.

To store: Pour the extract into ice cube trays – it fills approximately two trays, making about 20 cubes. Freeze overnight. Remove the cubes and store in a plastic bag; return to the freezer. Or simply pour into a container and freeze; you can break off chunks as you need them.

To use: Add a frozen chunk or one or more cubes of extract to recipes for soups, sauces, stews and casseroles. If your recipe calls for onions, defrost the extract first until it's soft enough to purée with the onion. This extracts the phenols from the onion, too. Then add to the dish.

Note: Quantities are approximate. Substitute your favourite herbs or blend.

SALAD DRESSINGS

VINAIGRETTE

*This tasty dressing uses olive oil, a heart-healthy fat,
and picks up extra prebiotics from the basil.*

For 240 ml of dressing, enough for approximately 8 servings of salad:

120 ml balsamic or red wine vinegar
120 ml extra virgin olive oil
1 teaspoon dried basil
2 teaspoons chopped spring onions
½ teaspoon whole grain or brown mustard (optional)
¼ teaspoon salt (or adjust to taste)

Put the vinegar, olive oil, basil, spring onions, mustard (if desired) and salt into a food processor or blender. Purée to make the vinaigrette. Use immediately or store in the refrigerator until needed. It will pour and taste best if used at room temperature.

YOGHURT RANCH DRESSING

*My kids love ranch dressing – and they've both given this version a
thumbs-up. It's richer in probiotics and prebiotics than ranch
dressings already mixed with buttermilk and sold in a bottle.*

For 240 ml of dressing, enough for approximately 8 servings of salad:

120 ml buttermilk
110 grams plain yoghurt
1 tablespoon extra virgin olive oil
½ teaspoon onion powder
¼ teaspoon garlic powder
¼ teaspoon salt
⅛ teaspoon dried dill
⅛ teaspoon black pepper
⅛ teaspoon dried celery seed
1 tablespoon parmesan (optional)

Mix buttermilk, yoghurt and olive oil. Stir in the onion powder, garlic powder, salt, dill, pepper, and celery seed. For parmesan ranch dressing, add parmesan.

This dressing can be stored in the refrigerator in a sealed container for about a week.

Note: If you normally use a prepared dry mix to make ranch dressing, that's okay, too. Usually the mix is added to a blend that's half mayonnaise and half buttermilk. Follow the directions, substituting plain yoghurt for the mayonnaise.

THOUSAND ISLAND YOGHURT DRESSING

This popular dressing completes a Reuben sandwich. It also can be used for other sandwiches and burgers, as well as for salads. My version of Thousand Island dressing substitutes yoghurt for the usual mayonnaise – cutting the fat while boosting the probiotics.

*For 360 grams, enough for about 24 sandwiches (about
1 tablespoon of dressing for each) or 12 portions of salad (about
2 tablespoons of dressing for each):*

150 grams plain low-fat yoghurt
3 tablespoons ketchup
2 tablespoons extra virgin olive oil
2 tablespoons Concord grape juice
2 hard-boiled eggs, finely chopped
1 tablespoon finely chopped green pepper
1 tablespoon finely chopped mild white onion
1 tablespoon finely chopped chives
pinch of salt (optional) or to taste

Mix together the yoghurt, ketchup, olive oil and grape juice. Stir in
the chopped eggs, pepper, onion and chives. Taste, and then add
salt if desired. If you prefer a creamy texture, purée the ingredients
in a food processor. The dressing can be served immediately or
refrigerated for up to a week.

Note: If you like, add more probiotics by substituting 2 tablespoons
of finely chopped fermented gherkins for the chopped green
pepper and chives.

SALADS

BEAN SALAD

*This is a variation of a dish that we tasted (and loved for
its fresh flavour) at a party given by friends. It can be served
as a side dish or with tortilla chips as a salsa. Leftovers are no
problem: the salad is even more tasty the next day.*

For 8 servings as a salad or side dish:

1 tin (340 to 454 grams) black beans, drained and rinsed
1 tin (340 to 454 grams) black-eyed peas, drained and rinsed
1 tin (340 to 454 grams) pinto beans, drained and rinsed
1 red pepper, chopped
1 green pepper, chopped
1 yellow pepper, chopped
1 red onion, chopped
230 grams shredded carrots
240 ml red wine vinegar
1 teaspoon extra virgin olive oil
60 ml Concord grape juice

Combine the black beans, black-eyed peas, pinto beans, red pepper, green pepper, yellow pepper, onion and carrots in a large mixing bowl. In a separate bowl or jug, mix together the vinegar, oil and grape juice. Pour over the vegetables. Serve immediately, or refrigerate overnight. It will taste even better the next day.

BLUE CHEESE, PEAR AND WALNUT SALAD

This delicious salad can be served as a lunch main course or as a small side salad. It is easy to make, flavoursome – and full of probiotics and prebiotics.

For 4 servings as a lunch main course; 8 servings as a side salad:

1 kilo salad greens, torn, washed and dried
230 grams walnut pieces (toasted or not toasted, as you prefer)
2 pears, cored and cubed but not peeled
110 to 230 grams Gorgonzola, blue or Roquefort cheese, crumbled
60 grams dried cranberries
120 ml vinaigrette dressing (see recipe on page 354)

Put the greens, walnuts, pear cubes, cheese and cranberries in a salad bowl. Pour the dressing over the salad and toss.

CREAMY WALDORF SALAD

Traditionally, Waldorf salad is made with apples, nuts, celery and mayonnaise. This version adds carrots and raisins, and substitutes a generous amount of yoghurt for the mayonnaise. The result is a delicious salad with more probiotics and prebiotics – and a lot less fat – than the traditional version.

For 4 to 6 servings:

Dressing:

> 230 grams low-fat plain yoghurt
> rind of 1 orange, grated
> 1 tablespoon honey
> pinch of salt

Salad:

> 80 grams pecans, coarsely chopped
> 2 large apples, unpeeled
> 2 stalks celery, chopped
> 2 carrots or 16 baby carrots, sliced into thin rounds
> 60 grams raisins
> 4 to 6 large lettuce leaves (one leaf per serving)

Prepare the dressing: In a medium bowl, mix together the yoghurt, orange rind, honey and salt.

Prepare the salad: Toast the pecans at 170°C for 10 minutes to intensify their flavour; set aside. Core and dice the apples; stir them into the yoghurt dressing to prevent them from browning. Stir in the chopped celery, sliced carrots and raisins. The salad can be refrigerated for several hours. Just before serving, stir in the toasted pecans.

To serve: Put a lettuce leaf on each plate. Top with a portion of salad.

Notes: If you're accustomed to mayonnaise, try substituting plain yoghurt for half of the mayonnaise in your usual recipe.

To save time, use 230 grams of lemon- or lime-flavoured yoghurt instead of the dressing in the recipe.

DIPS

GUACAMOLE

Okay, some people will argue that real guacamole isn't made with yoghurt. However, this creamy variation is a favourite with our guacamole-loving household and friends. Use it as a dip, as a tasty sandwich sauce – or even as a burger topping. It's great for making nachos, along with grated cheddar cheese and refried or black beans.

For 4 servings:

2 avocados
80 grams finely chopped onion
3 cloves garlic, peeled and minced
60 grams plain yoghurt
⅛ teaspoon salt
1 tablespoon lime juice (optional)
1 medium tomato, finely chopped (optional)

Cut each avocado in half, remove the stone, scoop out the inside of the avocado and add to a mixing bowl. Mash the avocados slightly with a fork or use a food processor. Add the chopped onion, garlic, yoghurt and salt, plus lime juice if desired. Continue to mash or purée the mixture until it reaches a smooth consistency. Stir in the chopped tomato if you wish.

CREAMY SALSA

A colleague told me about this incredibly quick and simple dip. To be honest, I didn't believe it could possibly taste that good – until I made it. Serve the salsa as a dip for tortilla chips or fresh vegetables: carrot or celery sticks, pepper strips, cucumber slices, broccoli or cauliflower florets. Or use it to top a jacket potato or Tex-Mex salad.

For 230 grams, enough for 4 to 8 servings as a dip, or 8 servings as a jacket potato topping or salad dressing:

110 grams salsa (see note)
110 grams plain yoghurt

Stir the salsa and yoghurt together. That's it!

Note: If you use a purchased salsa, check the label. Select a brand that lists the herbs and spices it contains. The flavour should come from these, not from 'natural flavours'. That term refers to flavouring ingredients that are usually derived from other foods and that don't contain valuable phenols.

SOUPS

CHICKEN-TORTILLA SOUP

This is a prebiotic-rich recipe that also includes probiotics. Yoghurt and cheese are added after the soup has been removed from the heat, to maximise their nutritional value and to give the dish a rich, creamy flavour. I like to serve the soup with a plate of extra tortilla chips, guacamole, creamy salsa and refried beans. A glass of Tea Sangria makes for an enjoyable Tex-Mex combination. (See recipes for Guacamole, Creamy Salsa and Tea Sangria.)

For 8 servings, each approximately 240 ml:

230 grams chopped onion

2 garlic cloves

2 teaspoons ground cumin

2 teaspoons chilli powder

60 ml red wine

1 tablespoon extra virgin olive oil

500 grams shredded or finely chopped cooked chicken breast

230 grams frozen sweetcorn

110 grams ground carrots

1 tin (110 to 170 grams) chopped green chilli peppers, undrained

2 tins (340 to 454 grams) chicken stock

1 tin (340 to 454 grams) chopped tomatoes, undrained

1 tin (340 to 454 grams) tomato sauce

1 teaspoon tamari or soya sauce

110 grams plain yoghurt

450 grams grated cheddar cheese

230 grams crushed baked tortilla chips

In a blender or food processor, purée the onion, garlic, cumin, chilli powder and red wine. Then add the olive oil and purée again. This flavouring mix can be used immediately, or you can prepare it ahead of time and refrigerate or freeze it.

To prepare the soup: into a pan that holds at least 3 litres, put the cooked chicken breast, sweetcorn, carrots, chopped chilli peppers, stock, chopped tomatoes, tomato sauce and tamari or soya sauce. Heat to near boiling, and then keep warm for at least 5 minutes (no need to boil). Add the flavouring mix.

Just prior to serving, remove the soup from the heat and stir in the yoghurt. Ladle soup into bowls. Top each portion with approximately 56 grams grated cheese and 2 tablespoons of crushed tortilla chips.

Notes: If you like black beans as much as I do, add 1 can (340 to 454 grams), drained, to this soup for both added flavour and fibre.

Use the same basic recipe to create a hearty, delicious black bean chilli, which is thicker than the soup – and meat-free. Just substitute 1 tin (340 to 454 grams) of black beans, drained, for the diced chicken and use 1 tin (340 to 454 grams) of vegetable stock instead of 2 tins of chicken stock.

TOMATO SOUP WITH PORRIDGE AND GARLIC

Who says that porridge is just for breakfast? This flavoursome and unusual soup is loaded with prebiotics – and it's quick and easy to prepare. In case you're wondering: the toasted rolled oats add flavour, but they look like bits of pasta. Unless you tell them, no one would guess it's porridge.

For 4 servings:

110 grams uncooked rolled oats (slow-cooking kind)
1 tablespoon olive oil
1 onion, finely chopped
3 large cloves garlic, minced
1 tin (400 to 454 grams) chopped tomatoes, undrained
700 ml vegetable or other stock

In a 2-litre saucepan, toast the rolled oats over a medium heat for about 3 to 5 minutes, shaking the pan or stirring to make sure they don't burn. Toasted oats will be fragrant and slightly dark. Pour them into a bowl and set aside.

Add the olive oil to the saucepan and tilt so that it coats the bottom. When the olive oil is hot, add the chopped onion and minced garlic. Cook for about 5 minutes, stirring occasionally. Add the chopped tomatoes and broth. Bring the soup to a simmer. Add the toasted porridge. Continue to simmer for about 10 minutes, stirring occasionally. Taste the soup and add salt if necessary.

MAIN DISHES

HEARTY MARINARA SAUCE WITH WHOLEWHEAT PASTA

At our house, this flavoursome tomato sauce is known as Dad's Secret Recipe. Served with wholewheat pasta, it's a family favourite – and it gets rave reviews from my kids' friends: 'This tastes just like pizza!' Little do they know that it's rich in prebiotics. (That's the secret.)

We often double the sauce recipe because it tastes even better the next day. We usually serve it over pasta, but also use it as a topping for rice. The sauce works for pizza, lasagne and chicken parmesan, too.

For 8 servings:

Marinara Sauce:

230 grams chopped onion

2 garlic cloves, chopped

1 tablespoon dried oregano

1 teaspoon dried basil

60 ml red wine

2 tablespoons extra virgin olive oil

1 tin (400 to 454 grams) tomato sauce

1 tin (340 to 454 grams) chopped tomatoes, undrained

1 tin or tube (170 grams) tomato paste

110 grams ground carrots

60 grams ground flaxseeds

2 heaped tablespoons refried beans (tinned or home-made)

60 ml Concord grape juice (or other dark berry juice)

1 teaspoon tamari soya sauce

Pasta:

500 grams dried wholewheat pasta

Toppings:

1 small bunch fresh oregano, finely chopped

500 grams grated cheese (parmesan, provolone or Gouda)

Make the sauce: In a blender or food processor, purée the onion, garlic, dried oregano, basil and red wine. Add the olive oil and purée again; set aside. This flavour blend can be prepared ahead of time and stored in the refrigerator or freezer.

In a saucepan that holds at least 2 litres, mix the tomato sauce, chopped tomatoes, tomato paste, ground carrots, flaxseeds, refried beans, juice and tamari. Cook over a medium heat, stirring occasionally, until the sauce is almost boiling. This takes about 5 minutes. Add the flavour blend that was set aside earlier.

Taste the sauce to check flavourings. If it's too acidic, add more juice. Alternatively, you can cut the acidity and make the sauce creamy by adding small amounts of plain yoghurt to taste.

While the sauce is heating, cook the pasta according to the directions on the packet.

Serve the pasta in individual dishes, topped with sauce. Sprinkle chopped fresh oregano and grated cheese on each serving.

Note: You can add meatballs, vegetarian meat substitutes or leftover diced chicken or turkey to the sauce. We sometimes add finely chopped fresh vegetables, such as green peppers or broccoli. Or we substitute fire-roasted for regular chopped tomatoes for a wonderful roasted flavour.

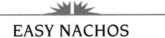

EASY NACHOS

My favourite comment from my son about eating a probiotic- and prebiotic-rich meal came in response to a plateful of nachos that I'd made him for dinner. 'Are these good for you?' he asked. 'Yes,' I told him. He gave me a big smile. 'Wow, this is great,' he said. 'I feel like I'm eating junk food.'

For 4 servings:

Refried bean sauce:

　　1 tin (340 to 454 grams) refried beans

　　1 tin (60 grams) diced green chilli peppers, drained

　　1 clove garlic, crushed

　　3 tablespoons finely chopped onion

　　3 tablespoons salsa (see note about salsa on page 360)

　　170 grams stone-ground corn chips (low-fat or baked)

　　110 grams aged cheddar cheese, grated

　　230 grams ground or grated carrots

　　1 kilo shredded lettuce

　　110 grams salsa

　　110 grams guacamole (optional)

　　2 tomatoes, diced (optional)

　　225 to 450 grams diced cooked chicken (optional)

Prepare the refried bean sauce: in a saucepan, mix together the refried beans, chilli peppers, garlic, onion and 3 tablespoons salsa. Heat until warm.

On each plate, spread a layer of corn chips and pour bean sauce over it. Sprinkle grated cheese on top of the bean sauce. Let it sit for a minute to soften the cheese. Add layers of carrots and lettuce, and top with the additional salsa plus any of the optional ingredients.

Note: Feel free to vary the quantity of corn chips, cheese, veggies and salsa.

SIDE DISHES

CHEESY GARLIC MASHED POTATOES

This is one of my daughter's favourite side dishes. I've adapted the recipe to maximise its probiotic and prebiotic content.

For 8 servings:

80 grams chopped onion

6 cloves garlic, peeled

2 teaspoons dried oregano, basil or Italian seasoning

60 ml white wine

2 tablespoons extra virgin olive oil

2 kilos diced, unpeeled baking potatoes (about 8 potatoes)

110 grams plain yoghurt

230 grams grated aged cheddar cheese

Purée the onion, garlic, oregano or other herbs and white wine in a food processor or blender. Then add the olive oil and purée again; set aside. This flavoursome onion-garlic blend can be made in advance and stored in the refrigerator or freezer; allow it to come to room temperature before using.

Put the unpeeled diced potatoes in a saucepan and cover with water. Bring to the boil and simmer until the potatoes are tender, approximately 5 to 10 minutes – check to make sure they're done.

Drain the potatoes, transfer to a mixing bowl and add the onion-garlic mix, yoghurt and grated cheese. Mash the potatoes with a fork or potato masher until smooth, or use a mixer at medium speed. Serve immediately or transfer the potatoes to an ovenproof dish and keep warm in the oven for up to an hour.

RAITA (INDIAN CUCUMBER YOGHURT SAUCE)

Raita is one of my favourite Indian dishes. It's a light-tasting side dish that complements any spicy main course – and it adds an appealing tang to grilled fish or prawns. Also use it as a sauce for rice or as a dip for pitta wedges or bread sticks. This version of raita – designed to maximise probiotic and prebiotic content – is loaded with nutrients.

For 480 ml, enough to serve 4 to 8 as a side dish:

230 grams plain yoghurt
1 teaspoon extra virgin olive oil
½ teaspoon cumin
⅛ teaspoon salt
1 unpeeled cucumber, finely chopped
80 grams finely diced red onion
2 tablespoons finely diced celery

Put the yoghurt into a mixing bowl. Stir in the olive oil, cumin and salt. Add the cucumber, onion and celery. The raita can be served immediately, but the flavour improves if it's refrigerated for an hour or more.

PUDDINGS

These recipes are not necessarily low in sugar and some aren't low in fat. But so what, they're puddings! However, even a dessert can have nutritional value – and all these do.

FRESH FRUIT CRUNCH

This recipe is based on an apple crumble recipe I've been using for years. Recently, I decided to use uncooked fruit, to enrich its phenol content. My family has given this new version rave reviews.

For 6 to 8 servings:

Crumble:

> 230 grams rolled oats, uncooked (use the slow-cooking kind)
> 110 grams whole wheat flour
> 110 grams flaxseed meal
> 110 grams packed light golden (soft) sugar
> ⅛ teaspoon salt
> 60 grams butter, softened

Fruit:

> 1 kilo of berries or diced unpeeled peaches, apples or pears
> 1 teaspoon cinnamon
> 230 grams vanilla yoghurt or frozen yoghurt (optional)

Prepare the crumble: combine oats, flour, flaxseed meal, light golden sugar and salt in a mixing bowl. Mix in softened butter until crumbly. Spread in an even layer on the bottom of a shallow baking dish about 25 cm by 15 cm. Bake at 175°C for 10 to 15 minutes, or until the oats are browned. Let the crumble cool in the baking dish. As the name suggests, it will be crumbly. You can make this topping in advance and store it in a sealed plastic bag or container, as you would store oatmeal biscuits.

To assemble, spoon the crumble into individual bowls. Cut up the fruit if you're using apples, peaches or pears. Place fruit on top of the crumble and sprinkle with cinnamon. Just before serving, top each portion with vanilla yoghurt or frozen yoghurt if desired.

FROZEN YOGHURT: GENERAL INSTRUCTIONS

Commercial frozen yoghurt rarely contains live probiotics. But if you own an ice cream maker, you can easily make probiotic-rich frozen yoghurt. Some ice cream makers are expensive, with built-in freezers and motors. But others are much simpler and cheaper. They rely upon your freezer to chill the mixture, and some require you to mix the ice cream yourself – a chore most kids are more than willing to do.

Any yoghurt smoothie recipe can be turned into frozen yoghurt – just put it in the ice cream maker and freeze it. You can also freeze low-fat flavoured yoghurt or kefir straight from the container. Be sure to check the capacity of your ice cream maker. You may need to make more than one batch.

BERRY FROZEN YOGHURT

For 6 servings:

500 grams fresh or frozen blueberries or strawberries
600 grams plain yoghurt
230 grams single cream
230 grams sugar

In a blender or food processor, purée the berries. Put the puréed berries, yoghurt, cream and sugar into a mixing bowl and stir until blended. Cover and refrigerate for at least 20 minutes. Freeze in an ice cream maker according to the manufacturer's directions.

CHOCOLATE YOGHURT SAUCE

A friend told me about this sauce. I was sceptical: I couldn't believe you could mix yoghurt, chocolate and cinnamon and get something that tasted good. But I was wrong. I love chocolate and this is excellent. Pour the sauce over fresh strawberries, frozen yoghurt, cakes or fruit crumble. Or just keep it in the fridge and grab a spoonful after dinner as a mini dessert. When it's chilled, the sauce is thick enough to make great chocolate-covered strawberries.

For 6 servings:

170 grams semi-sweet chocolate broken into pieces (or use chocolate chips)
170 grams plain low-fat yoghurt
½ teaspoon ground cinnamon

Put the chocolate into a bowl and melt over hot (not simmering) water, stirring constantly. When the chocolate has melted, remove it from the heat. Stir in the yoghurt and cinnamon until thoroughly blended. The sauce will be thick and creamy. If refrigerated, it thickens further and becomes mousse-like in consistency.

Note: Omit the cinnamon to get a more intense chocolate flavour. To make a chocolate mint sauce, use ½ teaspoon mint extract instead of cinnamon. If you prefer a sweeter chocolate sauce, use vanilla low-fat yoghurt instead of plain.

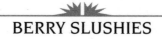
BERRY SLUSHIES

*This is a great chiller for a hot summer day. The only equipment
you need is a freezer, an ice cube tray and a blender. You can
make multiple batches of frozen juice cubes and store them in
plastic bags in the freezer. That way, you're ready to make
a slushie any time.*

For 2 servings:

420 ml berry juice (blueberry, cherry or a berry mix), divided
110 grams frozen berries (blueberries, strawberries, raspberries or a
   berry mix)

Pour 300 ml of juice into an ice cube tray and freeze. A typical ice
cube tray makes 30 ml ice cubes, so you'll have 10 juice cubes.

To make a slushie, put 10 juice cubes in the blender with the
remaining 120 ml of berry juice and the frozen berries. Cover the
blender and blend until smooth.

FROZEN SMOOTHIE WITH YOGHURT AND FRUIT

*This frozen smoothie makes a nutritious snack or pudding.
It's a delightful way to consume probiotics and prebiotics.
For convenience, make extra and keep a bag of
ready-to-blend yoghurt ice cubes in the freezer.*

For 1 serving:

170 to 230 grams low-fat vanilla yoghurt
110 grams frozen or fresh berries
60 ml milk

Spoon the yoghurt into an ice cube tray and freeze. You should have 6 to 8 cubes. To make a frozen smoothie, put the yoghurt cubes, berries and milk in a blender. Cover the blender and blend until smooth.

TROPICAL COFFEE SMOOTHIES

*A friend suggested this coffee-banana combination –
I never would have tried it on my own. I almost felt like a
kid on a dare the first time I tasted this smoothie. But to
my happy surprise, it was delicious. If you like frozen
coffee drinks, here's a healthy variation on the theme.*

For 2 servings:

170 to 230 grams low-fat vanilla yoghurt
1 ripe banana, sliced
120 ml milk
1 teaspoon instant coffee granules
2 tablespoons sugar

Freeze the yoghurt in an ice cube tray; you should have 6 to 8 cubes. To make a frozen smoothie, put the yoghurt cubes, sliced banana, milk, coffee granules and sugar in a blender. Cover and blend until smooth.

DRINKS

ICED TEA

*Iced tea is a popular drink in the USA in the summer time,
it is also is an incredible source of dietary phenols –
and so refreshing. It's my favourite beverage. I try to keep a jug
in my refrigerator at all times. If you have trouble with caffeine,
substitute tea that's been decaffeinated – preferably with
carbon dioxide (effervescent decaffeination) –
for all or some of the tea in this recipe.*

For 2 litres of tea, approximately 8 servings:

2 litres water
4 tea bags black tea
2 tea bags green tea

Put water in a saucepan and bring to a rolling boil. That's important because water must be near boiling to fully extract the dietary phenols from the tea leaves. Remove the saucepan from heat and add all the tea bags. Cover and let the tea bags steep for 5 to 15 minutes. That's enough time to extract the phenols. Because the water doesn't continue to boil during this period, phenol content stays high. (If the tea bags remain in the water for more than 15 minutes, the tea may become too bitter-tasting.)

The tea can be served as soon as the tea bags are removed – just pour it into an ice-filled glass. Add lemon or sugar if desired. If any tea is left over, transfer it to a jug or other container and refrigerate.

TEA COOLER

Use fruit juice – preferably one that's high in dietary phenols – to sweeten tea.

For 1 serving:

180 ml chilled tea
60 ml fruit juice (Concord grape, cherry, blueberry or pomegranate)

Pour the tea into a tall glass filled with ice. Add the fruit juice and stir.

TEA SANGRIA

This non-alcoholic sangria is a refreshing summer drink loaded with flavour and dietary phenols.

For 8 servings:

230 grams frozen raspberries
700 ml cold brewed tea
240 ml Concord grape juice
240 ml orange juice
480 ml tonic water
1 lemon, sliced
1 lime, sliced

Purée the raspberries in a blender and place in a jug that holds at least 2 litres. Add the tea, grape juice, orange juice and tonic water and stir. Put the sliced lemon and lime in the jug and stir again.

To serve: fill glasses with ice and pour the Tea Sangria over it. Put a slice of lemon and a slice of lime in each glass.

Note: Substitute other berry juices or pomegranate juice for the grape juice. To make a fizzier tea sangria, use 60 ml frozen Concord grape juice concentrate and 60 ml frozen orange juice concentrate instead of the grape and orange juice. Then increase the tonic water to 700 ml and the tea to 950 ml.

NOTES

Studies Cited in
The Probiotics Revolution

If you'd like to read any of the studies described in the book, you can find complete citations below. Studies are listed by the chapter and page that referred to them; some chapters are omitted because they don't mention particular studies. A full bibliography can be found on the book's website: http://www.probioticsrevolution.com.

To find abstracts – paragraph-long summaries of the studies – search PubMed (http://www.pubmed.com), a free service provided by the National Library of Medicine (NLM). See page 251 for instructions. Or check the websites of the journals, news services or organisations that published the articles.

Full-length versions of the articles are often available through the NLM or the journal websites. Sometimes they're free, but fees may be charged to read or download the complete text. Other options:

- **Use an Internet search engine to find the article.** Google Scholar (http://scholar.google.com) is often helpful.
- **Visit a library.** Your best bet is a medical school library, but ordinary

public libraries and college or university libraries often subscribe to major medical journals, too. If they don't have the journal you need, they may be able to obtain it for you via inter-library loan.

• **Write to the author.** Abstracts often contain contact information for making reprint requests.

Chapter 1

This introductory chapter briefly mentions studies that will be described later in the book. Citations to those studies are provided in the chapter in which the research is presented in more detail.

Page 3: The word is sometimes used in a limited way . . .
   2001. Health and Nutritional Properties of Probiotics in Food Including Powder Milk with Live Acid Bacteria. *Report of a Joint FOA/WHO Expert Consultation.*

Page 5: Indeed, the usual use of the term . . .
   Gibson, G. R. and M. B. Roberfroid. 1995 Dietary modulation of the human colonic microbiota: introducing the concept of prebiotics. *Journal of Nutrition 125:1401.*

Page 6: A fascinating Swedish study . . .
   Tubelius, P., V Stan and A. Zachrisson. 2005. Increasing work-place healthiness with the probiotic *Lactobacillus reuteri:* a randomised, double-blind placebo-controlled study. *Environmental Health 4:25.*

Page 18: Earlier, while a graduate student in my lab . . .
   Noverr, M. C., S. M. Phare, G. B. Toews, M. J. Coffey and G. B. Huffnagle. 2001. Pathogenic yeasts *Cryptococcus neoformans* and *Candida albicans* produce immunomodulatory prostaglandins. *Infection and Immunity 69:2957.*
   Noverr, M. C., G. B. Toews and G. B. Huffnagle. 2002. Production of prostaglandins and leukotrienes by pathogenic fungi. *Infection and Immunity 70:400.*

Page 19: After peer review, these exciting findings were published . . .
   Noverr, M. C., R. M. Noggle, G. B. Toews and G. B. Huffnagle. 2004. Role of antibiotics and fungal microbiota in driving pulmonary allergic responses. *Infection and Immunity 72:4996.*
   Noverr, M. C., N. R. Falkowski, R. A. McDonald, A. N. McKenzie and G. B. Huffnagle. 2005. Development of allergic airway disease in mice following antibiotic therapy and fungal microbiota increase: role of host genetics, antigen, and interleukin-13. *Infection and Immunity 73:30.*

Chapter 2

Page 42: Less well known is the fact that each of these changes . . .

Hambly, R. J., C. J. Rumney, J. M. Fletcher, P. J. Rijken and I. R. Rowland. 1997. Effects of high- and low-risk diets on gut microflora associated biomarkers of colon cancer in human flora-associated rats. *Nutrition and Cancer* 27:250.

Vargas, S. L., C. C. Patrick, G. D. Ayers and W. T. Hughes. 1993. Modulating effect of dietary carbohydrate supplementation on *Candida albicans* colonization and invasion in a neutropenic mouse model. *Infection and Immunity* 61:619.

Chapter 3

Page 55: According to a study published in the . . .

McCaig, L. F., R. E. Besser and J. M. Hughes. 2002. Trends in antimicrobial prescribing rates for children and adolescents. *Journal of the American Medical Association* 287:3096.

Page 55: In 2001, a study appeared . . .

McDonald, L. C., S. Rossiter, C. Mackinson, Y. Y. Wang, S. Johnson, M. Sullivan, R. Sokolow, E. DeBess, L. Gilbert, J. A. Benson, B. Hill and F. J. Angulo. 2001. Quinupristin-dalfopristin-resistant *Enterococcus faecium* on chicken and in human stool specimens. *New England Journal of Medicine* 345:1155.

Page 56: Two additional studies . . .

Sorensen, T. L., M. Blom, D. L. Monnet, N. Frimodt-Moller, R. L. Poulsen and F. Espersen. 2001. Transient intestinal carriage after ingestion of antibiotic-resistant *Enterococcus faecium* from chicken and pork. *New England Journal of Medicine* 345:1161.

White, D. G., S. Zhao, R. Sudler, S. Ayers, S. Friedman, S. Chen, P. F. McDermott, S. McDermott, D. D. Wagner and J. Meng. 2001. The isolation of antibiotic-resistant salmonella from retail ground meats. *New England Journal of Medicine* 345:1147.

Page 56: An Alarming Science Fair Project

Fackelmann, K. 2000. Drugs found in tap water. *USA Today*, 8 November.

Hartmann, A., A. C. Alder, T. Koller, and R. M. Widmer. 1998. Identification of fluoroquinone antibiotics as the main source of umuC genotoxicity in native hospital wastewater. *Environmental Toxicology and Chemistry* 17:377.

Page 57: Plain Soap and Water Is Still the Best

Aiello, A. E. and E. Larson. 2003. Antibacterial cleaning and hygiene products as an emerging risk factor for antibiotic resistance in the community. *Lancet Infectious Diseases* 3:501.

Page 58: According to a landmark CDC study . . .
Mannino, D. M., D. M. Homa, L. J. Akinbami, J. E. Moorman, C. Gwynn and S. C. Redd. 2002. Surveillance for asthma – United States, 1980–1999. *MMWR Surveillance Summary* 51:1.
1998. Worldwide variations in the prevalence of asthma symptoms: the International Study of Asthma and Allergies in Childhood (ISAAC). *European Respiratory Journal* 12:315.

Chapter 5

Page 92: A recent investigation in Germany . . .
De Vrese, M., P. Winkler, P. Rautenberg, T. Harder, C. Noah, C. Laue, S. Ott, J. Hampe, S. Schreiber, K. Heller and J. Schrezenmeir. 2005. Effect of *Lactobacillus gasseri* PA 16/8, *Bifidobacterium longum* SP 07/3, *B. bifidum* MF 20/5 on common cold episodes: a double blind, randomised, controlled trial. *Clinical Nutrition* 24:481.

Page 94: For example, some strains of the potentially . . .
Sperandio, V., A. G. Torres, B. Jarvis, J. P. Nataro and J. B. Kaper. 2003. Bacteria-host communication: the language of hormones. *Proceedings of the National Academy of Sciences USA* 100:8951.

Page 94: One of the first studies to link human stress . . .
Marcos, A., J. Warnberg, E. Nova, S. Gomez, A. Alvarez, R. Alvarez, J. A. Mateos and J. M. Cobo. 2004. The effect of milk fermented by yoghurt cultures plus *Lactobacillus casei* DN-114 001 on the immune response of subjects under academic examination stress. *European Journal of Nutrition* 43:381.

Page 99: Israeli researchers studied 261 formula-fed infants . . .
Weizman, Z., G. Asli and A. Alsheikh. 2005. Effect of a probiotic infant formula on infections in childcare centres: comparison of two probiotic agents. *Pediatrics* 115:5.

Page 100: The second study I want to tell you about . . .
Saavedra, J. M., A. Abi-Hanna, N. Moore and R. H. Yolken. 2004. Long-term consumption of infant formulas containing live probiotic bacteria: tolerance and safety. *American Journal of Clinical Nutrition* 79:261.

Page 102: A team in Turin, Italy, has conducted a series of investigations . . .
Savino, F., F. Cresi, S. Pautasso, E. Palumeri, V. Tullio, J. Roana,

L. Silvestro and R. Oggero. 2004. Intestinal microflora in breastfed colicky and non-colicky infants. *Acta Paediatrica* 93:825.

Savino, F., E. Palumeri, E. Castagno, F. Cresi, P. Dalmasso, F. Cavallo and R. Oggero. 2006. Reduction of crying episodes owing to infantile colic: a randomised controlled study on the efficacy of a new infant formula. *European Journal of Nutrition* 60:1304.

Savino, F., E. Castagno, R. Bretto, C. Brondello, E. Palumeri and R. Oggero. 2005. A prospective 10-year study on children who had severe infantile colic. *Acta Paediatrica (Supplement)* 94:129.

Page 103: For example, Finnish researchers recruited . . .
Hatakka, K., E. Savilahti, A. Ponka, J. H. Meurman, T. Poussa, L. Nase, M. Saxelin and R. Korpela. 2001. Effect of long term consumption of probiotic milk on infections in children attending day care centres: double blind, randomised trial. *British Medical Journal* 322:1327.

Page 104: At least five studies . . .
Hamilton-Miller, J. M. 2004. Probiotics and prebiotics in the elderly. *Postgraduate Medical Journal* 80:447.

Page 106: Italian investigators recruited adults over the age of . . .
Turchet, P., M. Laurenzano, S. Auboiron and J. M. Antoine. 2003. Effect of fermented milk containing the probiotic *Lactobacillus casei* DN-114001 on winter infections in free-living elderly subjects: a randomised, controlled pilot study. *Journal of Nutrition, Health and Ageing* 7:75.

Chapter 6

Page 114: An exciting pilot study of human patients . . .
Guslandi, M., P. Giollo and P. A. Testoni. 2003. A pilot trial of *Saccharomyces boulardii* in ulcerative colitis. *European Journal of Gastroenterology & Hepatology* 15:697.

Page 115: Two carefully conducted trials have shown that . . .
Mimura, T., F. Rizzello, U. Helwig, G. Poggioli, S. Schreiber, I. C. Talbot, R. J. Nicholls, P. Gionchetti, M. Campieri and M. A. Kamm. 2004. Once-daily high-dose probiotic therapy (VSL#3) for maintaining remission in recurrent or refractory pouchitis. *Gut* 53:108.

Gionchetti, P., F. Rizzello, A. Venturi, P. Brigidi, D. Matteuzzi, G. Bazzocchi, G. Poggioli, M. Miglioli and M. Campieri. 2000. Oral bacteriotherapy as maintenance treatment in patients with chronic pouchitis: a double-blind, placebo-controlled trial. *Gastroenterology* 119:305.

Page 121: For example, Irish investigators recruited . . .
O'Mahony, L., J. McCarthy, P. Kelly, G. Hurley, F. Luo, K. Chen, G. C. O'Sullivan, B. Kiely, J. K. Collins, F. Shanahan and E. M. Quigley. 2005.

Lactobacillus and *bifidobacterium* in irritable bowel syndrome: symptom responses and relationship to cytokine profiles. *Gastroenterology* 128:541.

Page 125: A 2004 study in the *American Journal of* . . .
Wang, K. Y., S. N. Li, C. S. Liu, D. S. Perng, Y. C. Su, D. C. Wu, C. M. Jan, C. H. Lai, T. N. Wang and W. M. Wang. 2004. Effects of ingesting *Lactobacillus*- and *Bifidobacterium*-containing yoghurt in subjects with colonised *Helicobacter pylori*. *American Journal of Clinical Nutrition* 80:737.

Page 126: For example, Czech investigators . . .
Sykora, J., K. Valeckova, J. Amlerova, K. Siala, P. Dedek, S. Watkins, J. Varvarovska, F. Stozicky, P. Pazdiora and J. Schwarz. 2005. Effects of a specially designed fermented milk product containing probiotic *Lactobacillus casei* DN-114 001 and the eradication of *H. pylori* in children: a prospective randomised double-blind study. *Journal of Clinical Gastroenterology* 39:692.

Page 127: For instance, investigators at several . . .
Guandalini, S., L. Pensabene, M. A. Zikri, J. A. Dias, L. G. Casali, H. Hoekstra, S. Kolacek, K. Massar, D. Micetic-Turk, A. Papadopoulou, J. S. de Sousa, B. Sandhu, H. Szajewska and Z. Weizman. 2000. *Lactobacillus* GG administered in oral rehydration solution to children with acute diarrhoea: a multicentre European trial. *Journal of Pediatric Gastroenterology and Nutrition* 30:54.

Page 129: In the Service of Science
Young, V. B. and T. M. Schmidt. 2004. Antibiotic-associated diarrhoea accompanied by large-scale alterations in the composition of the fecal microbiota. *Journal of Clinical Microbiology* 42:1203.

Page 130: According to a 2006 review article . . .
McFarland, L. V. 2006. Meta-analysis of probiotics for the prevention of antibiotic associated diarrhoea and the treatment of *Clostridium difficile* disease. *American Journal of Gastroenterology* 101:812.

Page 132: Probiotics – for Chickens!
Pascual, M., M. Hugas, J. I. Badiola, J. M. Monfort and M. Garriga. 1999. *Lactobacillus salivarius* CTC2197 prevents *Salmonella enteritidis* colonization in chickens. *Applied and Environmental Microbiology* 65:4981.

Chapter 7

Page 134: Beginning in the 1960s . . .
Mannino, D. M., D. M. Homa, L. J. Akinbami, J. E. Moorman, C. Gwynn and S. C. Redd. 2002. Surveillance for asthma – United States, 1980–1999. *MMWR Surveillance Summary* 51:1.

Page 135: In 1989, David Strachan . . .
Strachan, D. P. 1989. Hay fever, hygiene and household size. *British Medical Journal* 299:1259.

Page 136: Another group of researchers . . .
Gerrard, J. W., C. A. Geddes, P. L. Reggin, C. D. Gerrard and S. Horne. 1976. Serum IgE levels in white and Métis communities in Saskatchewan. *Annals of Allergy* 37:91.

Page 136: In a major British project, scientists analysed . . .
Sherriff, A. and J. Golding. 2002. Hygiene levels in a contemporary population cohort are associated with wheezing and atopic eczema in preschool infants. *Archives of Disease in Childhood* 87:26.

Page 136: In a review article on the subject . . .
Rook, G. A. and J. L. Stanford. 1998. Give us this day our daily germs. *Immunology Today* 19:113.

Page 137: As one solution to this dilemma . . .
Noverr, M. C. and G. B. Huffnagle. 2005. The 'microflora hypothesis' of allergic diseases. *Clinical and Experimental Allergy* 35:1511.

Page 137: In one particularly interesting study . . .
Bjorksten, B., P. Naaber, E. Sepp and M. Mikelsaar. 1999. The intestinal microflora in allergic Estonian and Swedish 2-year-old children. *Clinical and Experimental Allergy* 29:342.

Page 138: One of the largest such investigations . . .
McKeever, T. M., S. A. Lewis, C. Smith, J. Collins, H. Heatlie, M. Frischer and R. Hubbard. 2002. Early exposure to infections and antibiotics and the incidence of allergic disease: a birth cohort study with the West Midlands General Practice Research Database. *Journal of Allergy and Clinical Immunology* 109:43.

Page 139: One intriguing study . . .
Alm, J. S., J. Swartz, G. Lilja, A. Scheynius and G. Pershagen. 1999. Atopy in children of families with an anthroposophic lifestyle. *Lancet* 353:1485.

Page 141: Chinese investigators studied the benefits of yoghurt . . .
Wang, M. F., H. C. Lin, Y. Y. Wang and C. H. Hsu. 2004. Treatment of perennial allergic rhinitis with lactic acid bacteria. *Pediatric Allergy and Immunology* 15:152.

Page 142: A subsequent study by another team . . .
Peng, G. C. and C. H. Hsu. 2005. The efficacy and safety of heat-killed

Lactobacillus paracasei for treatment of perennial allergic rhinitis induced by house-dust mite. *Pediatric Allergy and Immunology* 16:433.

Page 142: Benefits aren't limited to children. . . .
Van de Water, J., C. L. Keen and M. E. Gershwin. 1999. The influence of chronic yoghurt consumption on immunity. *Journal of Nutrition* 129:1492S.

Page 148: In one very encouraging investigation . . .
Kalliomaki, M., S. Salminen, H. Arvilommi, P. Kero, P. Koskinen and E. Isolauri. 2001. Probiotics in primary prevention of atopic disease: a randomised placebo-controlled trial. *Lancet* 357:1076.

Page 149: Two other studies by the same team . . .
Kalliomaki, M., S. Salminen, T. Poussa, H. Arvilommi and E. Isolauri. 2003. Probiotics and prevention of atopic disease: 4-year follow-up of a randomised placebo-controlled trial. *Lancet* 361:1869.
Isolauri, E., T. Arvola, Y. Sutas, E. Moilanen and S. Salminen. 2000. Probiotics in the management of atopic eczema. *Clinical and Experimental Allergy* 30:1604.

Page 153: In one study, investigators at Seoul . . .
Kim, H., K. Kwack, D. Y. Kim and G. E. Ji. 2005. Oral probiotic bacterial administration suppressed allergic responses in an ovalbumin-induced allergy mouse model. *FEMS Immunology and Medical Microbiology* 45:259.

Page 153: In one of these investigations . . .
Majamaa, H. and E. Isolauri. 1997. Probiotics: a novel approach in the management of food allergy. *Journal of Allergy and Clinical Immunology* 99:179.
Viljanen, M., E. Savilahti, T. Haahtela, K. Juntunen-Backman, R. Korpela, T. Poussa, T. Tuure and M. Kuitunen. 2005. Probiotics in the treatment of atopic eczema/dermatitis syndrome in infants: a double-blind placebo-controlled trial. *Allergy* 60:494.

Chapter 8

Page 161: Microbes that normally live in the digestive tract don't necessarily . . .
Gardiner, G. E., C. Heinemann, A. W. Bruce, D. Beuerman and G. Reid. 2002. Persistence of *Lactobacillus fermentum* RC-14 and *Lactobacillus rhamnosus* GR-1 but not *L. rhamnosus* GG in the human vagina as demonstrated by randomly amplified polymorphic DNA. *Clinical and Diagnostic Laboratory Immunology* 9:92.
Reid, G., D. Charbonneau, J. Erb, B. Kochanowski, D. Beuerman,

R. Poehner and A. W. Bruce. 2003. Oral use of *Lactobacillus rhamnosus* GR-1 and *L. fermentum* RC-14 significantly alters vaginal flora: randomised, placebo-controlled trial in 64 healthy women. *FEMS Immunology and Medical Microbiology* 35:131.

Page 162: Though the evidence is not yet conclusive, some clinical . . .
Reid, G., A. W. Bruce, N. Fraser, C. Heinemann, J. Owen and B. Henning. 2001. Oral probiotics can resolve urogenital infections. *FEMS Immunology and Medical Microbiology* 30:49.

Page 165: The Cranberry Juice Option
Lynch, D. M. 2004. Cranberry for prevention of urinary tract infections. *American Family Physician* 70:2175.

Page 166: Those with low *Lactobacilli* counts . . .
Gupta, K., A. E. Stapleton, T. M. Hooton, P. L. Roberts, C. L. Fennell and W. E. Stamm. 1998. Inverse association of H_2O_2-producing *lactobacilli* and vaginal *Escherichia coli* colonization in women with recurrent urinary tract infections. *Journal of Infectious Diseases* 178:446.

Page 166: For example, Finnish investigators compared . . .
Kontiokari, T., J. Laitinen, L. Jarvi, T. Pokka, K. Sundqvist and M. Uhari. 2003. Dietary factors protecting women from urinary tract infection. *American Journal of Clinical Nutrition* 77:600.

Page 169: Studies find that people who form . . .
Sidhu, H., M. E. Schmidt, J. G. Cornelius, S. Thamilselvan, S. R. Khan, A. Hesse and A. B. Peck. 1999. Direct correlation between hyperoxaluria/oxalate stone disease and the absence of the gastrointestinal tract-dwelling bacterium *Oxalobacter formigenes*: possible prevention by gut recolonization or enzyme replacement therapy. *Journal of the American Society of Nephrology* 10(Suppl):S334.
Duncan, S. H., A. J. Richardson, P. Kaul, R. P. Holmes, M. J. Allison and C. S. Stewart. 2002. *Oxalobacter formigenes* and its potential role in human health. *Applied and Environmental Microbiology* 68:3841.
Troxel, S. A., H. Sidhu, P. Kaul and R. K. Low. 2003. Intestinal *Oxalobacter formigenes* colonization in calcium oxalate stone formers and its relation to urinary oxalate. *Journal of Endourology* 17:173.
Mittal, R. D., R. Kumar, H. K. Bid and B. Mittal. 2005. Effect of antibiotics on *Oxalobacter formigenes* colonization of human gastrointestinal tract. *Journal of Endourology* 19:102.

Page 169: Preliminary investigations in both animals and humans . . .
Campieri, C., M. Campieri, V. Bertuzzi, E. Swennen, D. Matteuzzi, S. Stefoni, F. Pirovano, C. Centi, S. Ulisse, G. Famularo and C. De Simone. 2001. Reduction of oxaluria after an oral course of lactic acid bacteria at high concentration. *Kidney International* 60:1097.

Sidhu, H., M. J. Allison, J. M. Chow, A. Clark and A. B. Peck. 2001. Rapid reversal of hyperoxaluria in a rat model after probiotic administration of *Oxalobacter formigenes. Journal of Urology 166:*1487.

Hoppe, B., G. von Unruh, N. Laube, A. Hesse and H. Sidhu. 2005. Oxalate degrading bacteria: new treatment option for patients with primary and secondary hyperoxaluria? *Urology Research 33:*372.

Lieske, J. C., D. S. Goldfarb, C. De Simone and C. Regnier. 2005. Use of a probiotic to decrease enteric hyperoxaluria. *Kidney International 68:1244.*

Chapter 9

Page 175: I'm intrigued by the fact that . . .

Stene, L. C. and P. Nafstad. 2001. Relation between occurrence of type 1 diabetes and asthma. *Lancet 357:*607.

Page 176: Faculty members at the University of Texas . . .

Hammer, R. E., S. D. Maika, J. A. Richardson, J. P. Tang and J. D. Taurog. 1990. Spontaneous inflammatory disease in transgenic rats expressing HLA-B27 and human beta 2m: an animal model of HLA-B27-associated human disorders. *Cell 63:1099.*

Page 178: In one investigation, scientists from . . .

Dieleman, L. A., M. S. Goerres, A. Arends, D. Sprengers, C. Torrice, F. Hoentjen, W. B. Grenther and R. B. Sartor. 2003. *Lactobacillus* GG prevents recurrence of colitis in HLA-B27 transgenic rats after antibiotic treatment. *Gut 52:370.*

Page 178: In an Italian study . . .

Calcinaro, F., S. Dionisi, M. Marinaro, P. Candeloro, V. Bonato, S. Marzotti, R. B. Corneli, E. Ferretti, A. Gulino, F. Grasso, C. De Simone, U. Di Mario, A. Falorni, M. Boirivant and F. Dotta. 2005. Oral probiotic administration induces interleukin-10 production and prevents spontaneous autoimmune diabetes in the non-obese diabetic mouse. *Diabetologia 48:1565.*

Page 180: They also support bacteria in our digestive . . .

Oberreuther-Moschner, D. L., G. Jahreis, G. Rechkemmer and B. L. Pool-Zobel. 2004. Dietary intervention with the probiotics *Lactobacillus acidophilus* 145 and *Bifidobacterium longum* 913 modulates the potential of human faecal water to induce damage in HT29clone19A cells. *British Journal of Nutrition 91:*925.

Page 182: Irish investigators conducted a study . . .

O'Mahony, L., M. Feeney, S. O'Halloran, L. Murphy, B. Kiely, J. Fitzgibbon, G. Lee, G. O'Sullivan, F. Shanahan and J. K. Collins. 2001.

Probiotic impact on microbial flora, inflammation and tumour development in IL-10 knockout mice. *Alimentary Pharmacology and Therapeutics* 15:1219.

Page 183: Do Antibiotics Increase Breast Cancer Risk?
Velicer, C. M., S. R. Heckbert, J. W. Lampe, J. D. Potter, C. A. Robertson and S. H. Taplin. 2004. Antibiotic use in relation to the risk of breast cancer. *Journal of the American Medical Association* 291:827.

Page 187: Studies with laboratory animals . . .
Fukushima, M. and M. Nakano. 1996. Effects of a mixture of organisms, *Lactobacillus acidophilus* or *Streptococcus faecalis* on cholesterol metabolism in rats fed on a fat- and cholesterol-enriched diet. *British Journal of Nutrition* 76:857.
Taranto, M. P., M. Medici, G. Perdigon, A. P. Ruiz Holgado and G. F. Valdez. 1998. Evidence for hypocholesterolemic effect of *Lactobacillus reuteri* in hypercholesterolemic mice. *Journal of Dairy Science* 81:2336.

Page 189: A team of scientists from the Institute for Genomic . . .
Gill, S. R., M. Pop, R. T. Deboy, P. B. Eckburg, P. J. Turnbaugh, B. S. Samuel, J. I. Gordon, D. A. Relman, C. M. Fraser-Liggett and K. E. Nelson. 2006. Metagenomic analysis of the human distal gut microbiome. *Science* 312:1355.

Page 190: Research in mice provides confirmation . . .
Backhed, F., H. Ding, T. Wang, L. V. Hooper, G. Y. Koh, A. Nagy, C. F. Semenkovich and J. I. Gordon. 2004. The gut microbiota as an environmental factor that regulates fat storage. *Proceedings of the National Academy of Sciences USA* 101:15718.
Ley, R. E., F. Backhed, P. Turnbaugh, C. A. Lozupone, R. D. Knight and J. I. Gordon. 2005. Obesity alters gut microbial ecology. *Proceedings of the National Academy of Sciences USA* 102:11070.
Turnbaugh, P. J., R. E. Ley, M. A. Mahowald, V. Magrini, E. R. Mardis and J. I. Gordon. 2006. An obesity-associated gut microbiome with increased capacity for energy harvest. *Nature* 444:1027.

Page 192: Tantalising Findings
Zemel, M. B., J. Richards, S. Mathis, A. Milstead, L. Gebhardt and E. Silva. 2005. Dairy augmentation of total and central fat loss in obese subjects. *International Journal of Obesity (London)* 29:391.

Page 193: A 2001 Columbia University survey . . .
Green, P. H. R., S. N. Stavropoulos, S. G. Panagi, S. L. Goldstein, D. J. McMahon, H. Absan and A. I. Neugut. 2001. Characteristics of adult coeliac disease in the USA: results of a national survey. *American Journal of Gastroenterology* 96:126.

Page 194: Recent studies suggest that the mucus layer . . .
Forsberg, G., A. Fahlgren, P. Horstedt, S. Hammarstrom, O. Hernell and M. L. Hammarstrom. 2004. Presence of bacteria and innate immunity of intestinal epithelium in childhood coeliac disease. *American Journal of Gastroenterology* 99:894.

Page 195: Scientists have learnt that a protein made by this yeast . . .
Nieuwenhuizen, W. F., R. H. Pieters, L. M. Knippels, M. C. Jansen and S. J. Koppelman. 2003. Is *Candida albicans* a trigger in the onset of coeliac disease? *Lancet* 361:2152.

Page 195: But according to preliminary studies, probiotics . . .
Nikawa, H., S. Makihira, H. Fukushima, H. Nishimura, Y. Ozaki, K. Ishida, S. Darmawan, T. Hamada, K. Hara, A. Matsumoto, T. Takemoto and R. Aimi. 2004. *Lactobacillus reuteri* in bovine milk fermented decreases the oral carriage of *mutans* streptococci. *International Journal of Food Microbiology* 95:219.
Caglar, E., N. Sandalli, S. Twetman, S. Kavaloglu, S. Ergeneli and S. Selvi. 2005. Effect of yoghurt with *Bifidobacterium* DN-173 010 on salivary *mutans* streptococci and lactobacilli in young adults. *Acta Odontologica Scandinavica* 63:317.

Page 197: One clue in support of that idea . . .
Aaron, L. A., M. M. Burke and D. Buchwald. 2000. Overlapping conditions among patients with chronic fatigue syndrome, fibromyalgia and temporomandibular disorder. *Archives of Internal Medicine* 160:221.
Cole, J. A., K. J. Rothman, H. J. Cabral, Y. Zhang and F. A. Farraye. 2006. Migraine, fibromyalgia and depression among people with IBS: a prevalence study. *BMC Gastroenterology* 6:26.

Page 197: It turns out that SIBO also could be a factor . . .
Pimentel, M., D. Wallace, D. Hallegua, E. Chow, Y. Kong, S. Park and H. C. Lin. 2004. A link between irritable bowel syndrome and fibromyalgia may be related to findings on lactulose breath testing. *Annals of the Rheumatic Diseases* 63:450.

Page 198: One promising hint comes from animal studies that . . .
Ait-Belgnaoui, A., W. Han, F. Lamine, H. Eutamene, J. Fioramonti, L. Bueno and V. Theodorou. 2006. *Lactobacillus farciminis* treatment suppresses stress induced visceral hypersensitivity: a possible action through interaction with epithelial cell cytoskeleton contraction. *Gut* 55:1090.
Verdu, E. F., P. Bercik, M. Verma-Gandhu, X. X. Huang, P. Blennerhassett, W. Jackson, Y. Mao, L. Wang, F. Rochat and S. M. Collins. 2006. Specific probiotic therapy attenuates antibiotic induced visceral hypersensitivity in mice. *Gut* 55:182.

Page 198: In one of these studies . . .

Kaartinen, K., K. Lammi, M. Hypen, M. Nenonen, O. Hanninen and A. L. Rauma. 2000. Vegan diet alleviates fibromyalgia symptoms. *Scandavian Journal of Rheumatology* 29:308.

Page 200: I've been following one fascinating hypothesis . . .

Bolte, E. R. 1998. Autism and *Clostridium tetani*. *Medical Hypotheses* 51:133.

Finegold, S. M., D. Molitoris, Y. Song, C. Liu, M. L. Vaisanen, E. Bolte, M. McTeague, R. Sandler, H. Wexler, E. M. Marlowe, M. D. Collins, P. A. Lawson, P. Summanen, M. Baysallar, T. J. Tomzynski, E. Read, E. Johnson, R. Rolfe, P. Nasir, H. Shah, D. A. Haake, P. Manning and A. Kaul. 2002. Gastrointestinal microflora studies in late-onset autism. *Clinical Infectious Diseases* 35:S6.

Parracho, H. M., M. O. Bingham, G. R. Gibson and A. L. McCartney. 2005. Differences between the gut microflora of children with autistic spectrum disorders and that of healthy children. *Journal of Medical Microbiology* 54:987.

Page 200: To further test Ellen Bolte's hypothesis . . .

Sandler, R. H., S. M. Finegold, E. R. Bolte, C. P. Buchanan, A. P. Maxwell, M. L. Vaisanen, M. N. Nelson and H. M. Wexler. 2000. Short-term benefit from oral vancomycin treatment of regressive-onset autism. *Journal of Child Neurology* 15:429.

Page 201: Investigators at the University of Reading . . .

Randerson, J. 2006. Study links autism to gut microbes. *Guardian Unlimited*, 4 September.

Chapter 10

Page 222: However, several recent reports suggest . . .

Tholstrup, T., C. E. Hoy, L. N. Andersen, R. D. Christensen and B. Sandstrom. 2004. Does fat in milk, butter and cheese affect blood lipids and cholesterol differently? *Journal of the American College of Nutrition* 23:169.

Page 222: While most research . . .

Bougle, D., N. Roland, F. Lebeurrier and P. Arhan. 1999. Effect of propionibacteria supplementation on fecal bifidobacteria and segmental colonic transit time in healthy human subjects. *Scandinavian Journal of Gastroenterology* 34:144.

Page 228: When *Health* magazine selected . . .

Raymond, J. 2006. World's healthiest foods. *Health*, March.

Chapter 11

Page 237: Guidance for Doctors
Floch, M. H., K. K. Madsen, D. J. Jenkins, S. Guandalini, J. A. Katz, A. Onderdonk, W. A. Walker, R. N. Fedorak and M. Camilleri. 2006. Recommendations for probiotic use. *Journal of Clinical Gastroenterology* 40:275.

Page 239: Similar doses have been used . . .
Gill, H. S., K. J. Rutherfurd, M. L. Cross and P. K. Gopal. 2001. Enhancement of immunity in the elderly by dietary supplementation with the probiotic *Bifidobacterium lactis* HN019. *American Journal of Clinical Nutrition* 74:833.

Page 239: Two doses of probiotics . . .
Szymanski, H., J. Pejcz, M. Jawien, A. Chmielarczyk, M. Strus and P. B. Heczko. 2006. Treatment of acute infectious diarrhoea in infants and children with a mixture of three *Lactobacillus rhamnosus* strains – a randomised, double-blind, placebo-controlled trial. *Alimentary Pharmacology and Therapeutics* 23:247.

Page 239: In a Danish investigation . . .
Rosenfeldt, V., E. Benfeldt, S. D. Nielsen, K. F. Michaelsen, D. L. Jeppesen, N. H. Valerius and A. Paerregaard. 2003. Effect of probiotic *Lactobacillus* strains in children with atopic dermatitis. *Journal of Allergy and Clinical Immunology* 111:389.

Page 241: A team of Polish and Swedish scientists . . .
Naruszewicz, M., M. L. Johansson, D. Zapolska-Downar and H. Bukowska. 2002. Effect of *Lactobacillus plantarum* 299v on cardiovascular disease risk factors in smokers. *American Journal of Clinical Nutrition* 76:1249.

Page 247: While it's possible that a generic . . .
ConsumerLab.com. 2006. Product Review: Probiotic Supplements (Including *Lactobacillus acidophilus*, *Bifidobacterium*, and Others). http://www.consumerlab.com.
Consumer Reports. 2005. Probiotics: are enough in your diet? *Consumer Reports*, July.

Chapter 15

Page 333: Research Support for the 'One Bite' Rule
Wardle, J., M. L. Herrera, L. Cooke and E. L. Gibson. 2003. Modifying children's food preferences: the effects of exposure and reward on acceptance of an unfamiliar vegetable. *European Journal of Clinical Nutrition* 57:341.

ABOUT THE AUTHORS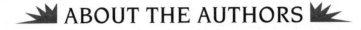

The website for *The Probiotics Revolution* is
www.probioticsrevolution.com

Gary B Huffnagle, PhD

Dr Huffnagle is a Professor of Internal Medicine (Pulmonary and
Critical Care Medicine) and Microbiology and Immunology at the
University of Michigan Medical School, one of the top ten medical
schools in the country. He also teaches an advanced undergraduate
microbiology course and a graduate-level immunology course at the
University of Michigan. He holds a BS in microbiology from
the Pennsylvania State University and a PhD in immunology
from the University of Texas Southwestern Medical School.

He has published over ninety articles about microbes and the immune system in peer-reviewed scientific journals, academic reviews and textbooks; his credentials also include more than sixty invited national and international lectureships. He holds or has held major grants from the National Heart, Lung and Blood Institute and the National Institute of Allergy and Infectious Diseases of the National Institutes of Health (NIH), including a grant from the NIH to further study the connection between digestive tract microbes and susceptibility to respiratory allergies.

His professional awards include a New Investigator Award from the Clinical Immunology Society, a Parker B. Francis Pulmonary Fellowship from the Francis Families Foundation and a New Investigator Award in Molecular Pathogenic Mycology from the Burroughs-Wellcome Fund. He serves or has served on editorial boards for the American Society for Microbiology (ASM) and the American Association of Immunologists (AAI), as well as on advisory panels for the National Institutes of Health.

Sarah Wernick

Ms Wernick is an award-winning freelance writer. Her books include the bestselling *Strong Women Stay Young* (Bantam, 1997 and 2000), written with Miriam Nelson of Tufts University, as well as *Strong Women Stay Slim* (Bantam, 1998). Among her other co-authored books is *Lung Cancer: Myths, Facts, Choices – and Hope* (Norton, 2003), written with Claudia Henschke, MD, of Cornell University and patient advocate Peggy McCarthy; the book received awards from the American Society of Journalists and Authors and the American Medical Writers Association. Her byline has appeared in *Woman's Day, Working Mother, Parents, Smithsonian*, the *New York Times* and many other magazines and newspapers. Her website is http://www.sarahwernick.com

INDEX

Read the Label!
Discover what's really in your food
Richard Emerson

The must-have guide to buying the finest, healthiest food for you and your family.

Do you know the difference between 'Use by' and 'Best before'? Or what is meant by 'Farmhouse' or 'Home-made'? And did you know that 75% of the salt we consume each day is added by food manufacturers during preparation or processing?

Read the Label! exposes the reality of food labelling and provides surprising information on how the facts can be manipulated. With an in-depth examination of the common ingredients found in our foods, information on how far you can trust the food label and clear guidance on how to make an informed decision about the products you buy, this book will change the way you shop forever.

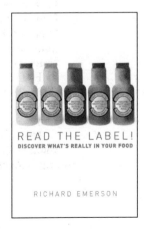

Solve Your Food Intolerance
A practical dietary programme to eliminate food intolerance
Dr John Hunter with Elizabeth Workman and Jenny Woolner

Many people are unaware that they suffer from food allergies or intolerance. Inexplicable rashes, a persistent runny nose, bloatedness, headaches and pronounced weight gain for no apparent reason are just some of the symptoms that may indicate a sensitivity to certain types of food.

Solve Your Food Intolerance is a practical dietary programme devised by one of the country's leading allergy specialists. It has been highly successful in combating a wide range of health problems, from Irritable Bowel Syndrome to eczema.

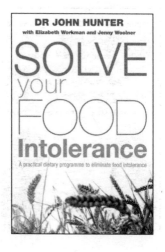

The Diet Doctors Inside and Out
The full body makeover plan that gets results
Dr Wendy Denning and Vicki Edgson

Diet Doctors Wendy Denning and Vicki Edgson can teach you to read your body's signals. What's your body trying to tell you?

The way you look and feel is largely dictated by what you eat. By learning to read your body's signs and making the necessary adjustments to your diet, you'll lose weight, sleep better, live longer and feel amazing. *The Diet Doctors Inside and Out* contains all the dietary and lifestyle advice you need for life-changing results.

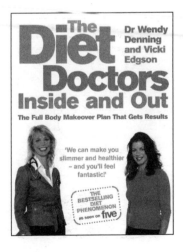

☐ Read the Label!	9780091917142	£5.99
☐ Solve Your Food Intolerance	9780091906658	£8.99
☐ The Diet Doctors Inside and Out	9780091910501	£12.99

FREE POSTAGE AND PACKING

Overseas customers allow £2.00 per paperback.

BY PHONE: 01624 677237

BY POST: Random House Books
c/o Bookpost, PO Box 29, Douglas
Isle of Man, IM99 1BQ

BY FAX: 01624 670923

BY EMAIL: bookshop@enterprise.net

Cheques (payable to Bookpost) and credit cards accepted.

Prices and availability subject to change without notice.
Allow 28 days for delivery.
When placing your order, please mention if you do not wish to receive any additional information.

www.rbooks.co.uk